A FEAST OF INFORMATION—
for people who love to eat but need to know
the calorie count of their meals.
BARBARA KRAUS 1989 CALORIE GUIDE
TO BRAND NAMES AND BASIC FOODS
lists thousands of basic and ready-to-eat
foods from appetizers to desserts—carry it to the
supermarket, to the restaurant, to the beach, to
the coffee cart, and on trips.
Flip through these fact-filled pages. Mix, match,
and keep track of calories as they add up. But
remember, strawberry shortcake is fattening any
way you slice it!

BARBARA KRAUS
1989 Calorie Guide
to
Brand Names and
Basic Foods

Barbara Kraus
1989 Calorie Guide to Brand Names and Basic Foods

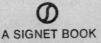

A SIGNET BOOK

NEW AMERICAN LIBRARY

For Keisuke Haruguchi & Family

Excerpted from *Dictionary of Calories and Carbohydrates*

SIGNET, SIGNET CLASSIC, MENTOR, ONYX, PLUME,
MERIDIAN AND NAL BOOKS
are published by NAL PENGUIN INC.,
1633 Broadway, New York, New York 10019

FIRST PRINTING, JANUARY, 1989

1 2 3 4 5 6 7 8 9

PRINTED IN THE UNITED STATES OF AMERICA

Foreword

The composition of the foods we eat is not static: it changes from time to time. In the case of *brand-name* products, manufacturers alter their recipes to reflect the availability of ingredients, advances in technology, or improvements in formulae. Each year new products appear on the market and some old ones are discontinued.

On the other hand, information on *basic foods* such as meats, vegetables, and fruits may also change as a result of the development of better analytical methods, different growing conditions, or new marketing practices. These changes, however, are usually relatively small as compared with those in manufactured products.

Some differences may be found between the values in this book and those appearing on the product labels. This is usually due to the fact that the Food and Drug Administration permits manufacturers to round the figures reported on labels. The data in this book are reported as calculated without rounding. If large differences between the two sets of values are noted, they may be due to changes in product formulae, and in those cases the label data should be used.

For all these reasons, a book of calorie or nutritive values of foods must be kept up to date by a periodic reviewing and revision of the data presented.

Therefore, this handy calorie counter will provide each year the most current and accurate estimates available. Generous use of this little book will help you and your family to select the right foods and the proper number of calories each member requires to gain, lose, or maintain healthy and attractive weight.

Barbara Kraus

Why This Book?

Some of the data presented here can be found in more detail in my bestselling *Calories and Carbohydrates,* a dictionary of 8,000 brand names and basic foods. Complete as it is, it is meant to be used as a reference book at home or in the office and not to be squeezed into a suit jacket or evening bag—it's just too big.

Therefore, responding to the need for a portable calorie guide, and one which can reflect food changes often, I have written this smaller and handier version. The selection of material and the additional new entries provide readers with pertinent data on thousands of products that they would prepare at home to take to work, eat in a restaurant or luncheonette, nibble on from the coffee cart, take to the beach, buy in the candy store, etcetera.

For the sake of saving space and providing you with a greater selection of products, I had to make certain compromises: whereas in the giant book there are several physical descriptions of a product, here there is but one.

For Beginners Only

The language of dieting is no more difficult to learn than any other new subject; in many respects, it's much easier, particularly if you restrict your education to clearly defined goals.

For you who never before had the need or the interest in a lesson in weight control, I offer the following elementary introduction, applicable to any diet, self-initiated or suggested by your doctor, nutritionist, or dietician.

A Calorie

An analysis of foods in terms of calories is most often the chosen method to describe the relative energy yielded by foods.

A calorie is a shorthand way to summarize the units of energy contained in any foodstuff or alcoholic beverage, similar to the way a thermometer indicates heat. One pound of fat is equal to 3,500 calories. Add this number of calories to those you need to balance your energy requirements and you will gain one pound; subtract it and you will lose a pound.

Other Nutrients

Carbohydrates—which include sugars, starches, and acids—are only one of several chemical compounds in foods that yield calories. Proteins, found mainly in beef, poultry, and fish; fats, found in oils, butter, marbling of meat, poultry skin; and alcohol, found in some beverages, also contribute calories. Except for alcohol, most foods contain at least some of these nutrients.

The amount of carbohydrates varies from zero in meats and a trace in alcohol to a heavy concentration in sugar, syrups, some fruits, grains, and root vegetables.

As of this date, the most respected nutritional researchers insist that some carbohydrate is necessary every day for maintaining good health. The amount to be included is an individual matter, and in any drastic effort to change your eating patterns, be sure to consult your doctor first.

Now, on how to use this new language.

To begin with, you use this book like a dictionary. If your plan is to cut down on calories, the easiest way to do so is to consult the portable calorie counter and keep an accurate count of your total intake of food and beverages for a period of seven days. If you have not gained or lost weight during that week, divide that number by seven and you'll have your maintenance diet expressed in calories. To lose weight, you must reduce your daily or weekly intake of calories below this maintenance level. (To gain, increase the intake.)

Keeping in mind that you want to stay healthy and eat well-balanced meals (which include the basic food groups: milk or milk products; meat, poultry, or fish; vegetables and fruits; and whole grain or enriched breads or cereals, as well as some fats or oils), you then start to cut down on your portion in order to reduce your intake of calories. There are many imaginative ways to diet without total withdrawal from one's favorite foods.

Once you know and don't have to guess what calories are in your foods, you can relax and enjoy them. It could turn out that dieting isn't so bad after all.

ABBREVIATIONS AND SYMBOLS

* = prepared as package directs[1]
< = less than
& = and
″ = inch
canned = bottles or jars as well as cans
dia. = diameter
fl. = fluid
liq. = liquid
lb. = pound
med. = medium

oz. = ounce
pkg. = package
pt. = pint
qt. = quart
sq. = square
T. = tablespoon
Tr. = trace
tsp. = teaspoon
wt. = weight

Italics or name in parentheses = registered trademark, ®. All data not identified by company or trademark are based on material obtained from the United States Department of Agriculture or Health, Education and Welfare/Food and Agriculture Organization.

EQUIVALENTS

By Weight	By Volume
1 pound = 16 ounces	1 quart = 4 cups
1 ounce = 28.35 grams	1 cup = 8 fluid ounces
3.52 ounces = 100 grams	1 cup = ½ pint
	1 cup = 16 tablespoons
	2 tablespoons = 1 fluid ounce
	1 tablespoon = 3 teaspoons
	1 pound butter = 4 sticks or 2 cups

---

[1]If the package directions call for whole or skim milk, the data given here are for whole milk unless otherwise stated.

A

Food and Description	Measure or Quantity	Calories
ABALONE, canned	4 oz.	91
AC'CENT	¼ tsp.	3
ALBACORE, raw, meat only	4 oz.	201
ALLSPICE (French's)	1 tsp.	6
ALMOND:		
In shell	10 nuts	60
Shelled, raw, natural, with skins	1 oz.	170
Roasted, dry (Planters)	1 oz.	170
Roasted, oil (Tom's)	1 oz.	180
ALMOND EXTRACT (Durkee) pure	1 tsp.	13
ALPHA-BITS, cereal (Post)	1 cup (1 oz.)	113
AMARETTO DI SARONNO	1 fl. oz.	83
ANCHOVY, PICKLED, canned, flat or rolled, not heavily salted, drained (Granadaisa)	2-oz. can	80
ANISE EXTRACT (Durkee) imitation	1 tsp.	16
ANISETTE:		
(DeKuyper)	1 fl. oz.	95
(Mr. Boston)	1 fl. oz.	88
APPLE:		
Fresh, with skin	2½″ dia.	61
Fresh, without skin	2½″ dia.	53
Canned (Comstock):		
Rings, drained	1 ring	30
Sliced	⅙ of 21-oz. can	45
Dried:		
(Del Monte)	1 cup	140
(Sun-Maid/Sunsweet)	2-oz. serving	150
Frozen, sweetened	1 cup	325
APPLE BROWN BETTY	1 cup	325
APPLE BUTTER (Smucker's) cider	1 T.	38
APPLE CHERRY BERRY DRINK, canned (Lincoln)	6 fl. oz.	90
APPLE CIDER:		
Canned:		
(Mott's) sweet	½ cup	59
(Tree Top)	6 fl. oz.	90
*Mix, *Country Time*	8 fl. oz.	98
APPLE-CRANBERRY DRINK (Hi-C):		
Canned	6 fl. oz.	90
*Mix	6 fl. oz.	72
APPLE-CRANBERRY JUICE, canned (Lincoln)	6 fl. oz.	100

Food and Description	Measure or Quantity	Calories
APPLE DRINK:		
Canned:		
Capri Sun, natural	6¾ fl. oz.	90
(Hi-C)	6 fl. oz.	92
*Mix (Hi-C)	6 fl. oz.	72
APPLE DUMPLINGS, frozen		
(Pepperidge Farm)	1 dumpling	260
APPLE, ESCALLOPED, frozen		
(Stouffer's)	4 oz.	140
APPLE-GRAPE JUICE, canned:		
(Musselman's)	6 fl. oz.	82
(Red Cheek)	6 fl. oz.	69
APPLE JACKS, cereal (Kellogg's)	1 cup (1 oz.)	110
APPLE JAM (Smucker's)	1 T.	53
APPLE JELLY:		
Sweetened (Smucker's)	1 T.	67
Dietetic:		
(Estee; Featherweight;		
Louis Sherry)	1 T.	6
(Diet Delight)	1 T.	12
APPLE JUICE:		
Canned:		
(Lincoln)	6 fl. oz.	90
(Musselman's)	6 fl. oz.	80
(Ocean Spray)	6 fl. oz.	90
(Red Cheek)	6 fl. oz.	85
(Thank You Brand)	6 fl. oz.	82
(Tree Top) regular	6 fl. oz.	90
Chilled (Minute Maid)	6 fl. oz.	100
*Frozen:		
(Minute Maid)	6 fl. oz.	100
(Seneca Foods) Vitamin C added	6 fl. oz.	90
(Tree Top)	6 fl. oz.	90
APPLE JUICE DRINK, canned		
(Sunkist)	8.5 fl. oz.	140
APPLE PIE (See PIE, Apple)		
APPLE RAISIN CRISP, cereal		
(Kellogg's)	⅔ cup	130
APPLE SAUCE:		
Regular:		
(A&P) regular	½ cup	110
(Comstock)	½ cup	100
(Del Monte)	½ cup	90
(Mott's):		
Natural style	½ cup	115
With ground cranberries	½ cup	110
(Musselman's)	½ cup	96
(Thank You Brand)	½ cup	87
(Tree Top) Natural	½ cup	60
Dietetic:		
(Del Monte, Lite; Diet Delight)	½ cup	50
(S&W) *Nutradiet,* white		
or blue label	½ cup	55

Food and Description	Measure or Quantity	Calories
(Thank You Brand)	½ cup	54
APPLE STRUDEL, frozen (Pepperidge Farm)	3 oz.	240
APRICOT:		
Fresh, whole	1 apricot	18
Canned, regular pack:		
(Del Monte) whole, or halves, peeled	½ cup	200
(Stokely-Van Camp)	1 cup	220
Canned, dietetic, solids & liq.:		
(Del Monte) Lite	½ cup	64
(Diet Delight):		
Juice pack	½ cup	60
Water pack	½ cup	35
(Featherweight):		
Juice pack	½ cup	50
Water pack	½ cup	35
(Libby's) Lite	½ cup	60
(S&W) *Nutradiet:*		
Halves, white or blue label	½ cup	50
Whole, juice	½ cup	40
Dried:		
(Del Monte; Sun-Maid; Sunsweet)	2 oz.	140
APRICOT & PINEAPPLE PRESERVE OR JAM:		
Sweetened (Smucker's)	1 T.	53
Dietetic:		
(Diet Delight; Louis Sherry)	1 T.	6
(S&W) *Nutradiet*	1 T.	12
APRICOT LIQUEUR (DeKuyper)	1 fl. oz.	82
APRICOT NECTAR:		
(Del Monte)	6 fl. oz.	100
(Libby's)	6 fl. oz.	110
APRICOT-PINEAPPLE NECTAR, canned, dietetic (S&W) *Nutradiet*, blue label	6 oz.	35
APRICOT PRESERVE, dietetic (Estee)	1 T.	6
ARBY'S:		
Bac'n Cheddar Deluxe	1 sandwich	561
Beef & Cheddar Sandwich	1 sandwich	490
Chicken breast sandwich	7¼-oz. sandwich	592
Croissant:		
Bacon & egg	1 croissant	420
Butter	1 croissant	220
Chicken salad	1 croissant	460
Ham & Swiss	1 croissant	330
Mushroom & Swiss	1 croissant	340
Sausage & egg	1 croissant	530
French fries	1½-oz. serving	211
Ham 'N Cheese	1 sandwich	353
Potato cakes	2 pieces	201

Food and Description	Measure or Quantity	Calories
Potato, stuffed:		
Broccoli & cheddar	1 potato	541
Deluxe	1 potato	648
Mushroom & cheese	1 potato	506
Taco	1 potato	619
Roast Beef:		
Regular	5 oz.	353
Junior	3 oz.	218
King	6.7 oz.	467
Super	9¼ oz.	501
Garden salad (no dressing)	1 serving	165
Chef's salad (no dressing)	1 serving	235
Cashew chicken salad (contains dressing)	1 serving	505
Crackers	1 packet	25
Croutons	1 packet	70
Dressings:		
Blue cheese	1 packet	390
Buttermilk	1 packet	460
Honey French	1 packet	350
Light Italian	1 packet	25
ARTICHOKE:		
Boiled	15-oz. artichoke	187
Canned (Cara Mia) marinated, drained	6-oz. jar	175
Frozen (Birds Eye) deluxe	⅓ pkg.	39
ASPARAGUS:		
Boiled	1 spear (½" dia. at base)	3
Canned, regular pack, solid & liq.:		
(Del Monte) spears, green or white	½ cup	20
(Green Giant)	8-oz. can	46
Canned, dietetic, solids & liq.:		
(Diet Delight)	½ cup	16
(Featherweight) cut spears	1 cup	40
(S&W) *Nutradiet*	1 cup	40
Frozen:		
(Birds Eye):		
Cuts	⅓ pkg.	29
Spears, regular or jumbo deluxe	⅓ pkg.	30
(Frosty Acres)	3.3 oz.	25
(Green Giant) cuts, butter sauce	3 oz.	57
(McKenzie)	⅓ pkg.	25
(Stouffer's) souffle	⅓ pkg.	115
ASPARAGUS PUREE, canned		
(Larsen)	½ cup	22
AUNT JEMIMA SYRUP (See SYRUP)		
AVOCADO, all varieties	1 fruit (10.7 oz.)	378
AWAKE (Birds Eye)	6 fl. oz.	84
AYDS:		
Butterscotch	1 piece	27
Chocolate, chocolate mint, vanilla	1 piece	26

4

B

Food and Description	Measure or Quantity	Calories
BACON, broiled:		
(Hormel) *Black Label*	1 slice	30
(Oscar Mayer):		
Regular slice	6-gram slice	35
Center cut	1 slice	24
Thick slice	1 slice	64
BACON BITS:		
Bac*Os (Betty Crocker)	1 tsp.	13
(French's) imitation	1 tsp.	6
(Hormel)	1 tsp.	10
(Libby's) crumbles	1 tsp.	8
(Oscar Mayer) real	1 tsp.	7
BACON, CANADIAN, unheated:		
(Eckrich)	1 oz.	35
(Hormel):		
Regular	1 slice	45
Light & Lean	1 slice	17
(Oscar Mayer) 93% fat free:		
Thin	.7-oz. slice	30
Thick	1-oz. slice	35
BACON, SIMULATED, cooked:		
(Oscar Mayer) *Lean'N Tasty*:		
Beef	1 strip	46
Pork	1 strip	54
(Swift's) *Sizzlean*, pork	1 strip	35
BAGEL (Lender's):		
Plain:		
Regular	1 bagel	150
Bagelette	1 bagel	70
Egg	1 bagel	150
Onion	1 bagel	160
Poppy seed	1 bagel	160
Raisin & honey	1 bagel	200
BAKING POWDER:		
(Calumet)	1 tsp.	2
(Davis)	1 tsp.	7
(Featherweight) low sodium, cereal free	1 tsp.	8
BAMBOO SHOOTS:		
Raw, trimmed	4 oz.	31
Canned, drained (Chun King)	½ cup	32
BANANA, medium (Dole)	6.3-oz. banana (weighed unpeeled)	101
BANANA EXTRACT (Durkee) imitation	1 tsp.	15

5

Food and Description	Measure or Quantity	Calories
BANANA NECTAR (Libby's)	6 fl. oz.	60
BANANA PIE (See PIE, Banana)		
BARBECUE SEASONING		
(French's)	1 tsp.	6
BARBERA WINE (Louis M.		
Martini) 12½% alcohol	3 fl. oz.	66
BARLEY, pearled (Quaker Scotch)	¼ cup	172
BASIL (French's)	1 tsp.	3
BASS:		
Baked, stuffed	3½" × 4½" × 1½"	531
Oven-fried	8¾" × 4½" × ⅝"	392
BAY LEAF (French's)	1 tsp.	5
B & B LIQUEUR	1 fl. oz.	94
B.B.Q. SAUCE & BEEF, frozen		
(Banquet) *Cookin' Bag,* sliced	4-oz. serving	133
BEAN, BAKED:		
(USDA):		
With pork & molasses sauce	1 cup	382
With pork & tomato sauce	1 cup	311
Canned:		
(Allens) *Wagon Master*	1 cup	260
(B&M) *Brick Oven*:		
Pea bean with pork in brown		
sugar sauce	8 oz.	300
Red kidney bean in brown		
sugar sauce	8 oz.	290
Vegetarian	8 oz.	250
(Campbell):		
Home style	8-oz. can	270
With pork & tomato sauce	8-oz. can	240
(Friend's):		
Pea	9-oz. serving	360
Yellow eye	9-oz. serving	360
(Furman's) & pork, in tomato		
sauce	8 oz.	245
(Grandma Brown's)	8 oz.	289
(Hormel) *Short Orders,* with		
bacon	7½-oz. can	330
BEAN, BARBECUE (Campbell)	7⅞-oz. can	678
BEAN & BEEF BURRITO DINNER,		
frozen (Swanson)	15¼-oz. dinner	720
BEAN, BLACK OR BROWN:		
Dry	1 cup	678
Canned (Goya) black	1 cup.	250
BEAN, FAVA, canned (Progresso)	4 oz.	90
BEAN & FRANKFURTER, canned:		
(Campbell) in tomato and molasses		
sauce	7⅞-oz. can	360
(Hormel) *Short Orders*, 'n wieners	7½-oz. can	280
BEAN & FRANKFURTER		
DINNER, frozen:		
(Banquet)	10¼-oz. dinner	500

Food and Description	Measure or Quantity	Calories
(Swanson)	12½-oz. dinner	550
BEAN, GARBANZO, canned:		
Regular (*Old El Paso*)	½ cup	77
Dietetic (S&W) *Nutradiet,* low sodium, green label	½ cup	105
BEAN, GREEN:		
Boiled, 1½" to 2" pieces, drained	½ cup	17
Canned, regular pack, solids & liq.:		
(Allen's):		
Whole	½ cup	21
With dry shelled beans	½ cup	40
(Comstock)	½ cup	25
(Del Monte)	4 oz.	20
(Green Giant) French or whole	½ cup	21
(Sunshine)	½ cup	20
Canned, dietetic, solids & liq.:		
(Del Monte) No Salt Added	4 oz.	19
(Diet Delight; S&W, *Nutradiet*)	½ cup	20
(Larsen) *Fresh-Lite*	½ cup	20
Frozen:		
(Birds Eye):		
Cut or French	⅓ pkg.	30
French, with almonds	⅓ pkg.	34
Whole, deluxe	⅓ pkg.	26
(Frosty Acres)	3 oz.	25
(Green Giant):		
Cut or French, with butter sauce	½ cup	40
Cut, *Harvest Fresh*	½ cup	25
(Seabrook Farms; Southland)	⅓ pkg.	29
BEAN, GREEN & MUSHROOM CASSEROLE (Stouffer's)	½ pkg.	150
BEAN, GREEN, WITH POTATOES, canned (Sunshine) solids & liq.	½ cup	34
BEAN, ITALIAN:		
Canned (Del Monte) solids & liq.	4 oz.	25
Frozen (Birds Eye)	⅓ pkg.	38
BEAN, KIDNEY:		
Canned, regular pack, solids & liq.		
(Allen's) red	½ cup	110
(Comstock)	½ cup	120
(Furman) red, fancy, light	½ cup	121
(Goya);		
Red	½ cup	115
White	½ cup	100
(Progresso)	½ cup	95
(Van Camp):		
Light	8 oz.	194
New Orleans style	8 oz.	188
Red	8 oz.	213
Canned, dietetic (S&W) *Nutradiet,* low sodium,	½ cup	90

Food and Description	Measure or Quantity	Calories
BEAN, LIMA:		
Boiled, drained	½ cup	94
Canned, regular pack, solids & liq.:		
(Allen's):		
Regular	½ cup	60
Baby butter	½ cup	55
(Del Monte)	4 oz.	70
(Furman's)	½ cup	92
(Sultana) butter bean	¼ of 15-oz. can	82
Canned, dietetic (Featherweight)	½ cup	80
Frozen:		
(Birds Eye) baby	⅓ pkg.	130
(Frosty Acres):		
Baby	3.3 oz.	130
Butter	3.2 oz.	140
Fordhook	3.3 oz.	100
(Green Giant):		
In butter sauce	½ cup	120
Harvest Fresh or polybag	½ cup	100
(Seabrook Farms):		
Baby lima	⅓ pkg.	126
Baby butter bean	⅓ pkg.	139
Fordhooks	⅓ pkg.	98
BEAN, PINK, canned		
(Goya)	½ cup	115
BEAN, PINTO (Goya)	½ cup	100
BEAN, RED, canned		
(Goya)	½ cup	79
BEAN, REFRIED, canned:		
Old El Paso:		
Plain	4 oz.	106
With sausage	4 oz.	224
(Ortega) lightly spicy or true bean	½ cup	170
BEAN, ROMAN,		
canned (Goya)	½ cup	81
BEAN SALAD, canned		
(Green Giant)	¼-oz. serving	80
BEAN SOUP (See SOUP, Bean)		
BEAN SPROUT:		
Mung, raw	½ lb.	80
Mung, boiled, drained	¼ lb.	32
Soy, raw	½ lb.	104
Soy, boiled, drained	¼ lb.	43
Canned (Chun King)	4 oz.	40
BEAN, WHITE, canned		
(Goya) solids & liq.	½ cup	105
BEAN, YELLOW OR WAX:		
Boiled, 1″ pieces, drained	½ cup	18
Canned, regular pack, solids & liq.:		
(Comstock)	½ cup	20
(Del Monte) cut or french	½ cup	18

Food and Description	Measure or Quantity	Calories
(Libby's) cut	4 oz.	23
(Stokley-Van Camp)	½ cup	23
Canned, dietetic (Featherweight) cut, solids & liq.	½ cup	25
Frozen (Frosty Acres)	3 oz.	25
BEEF, choice grade, medium done:		
Brisket, braised:		
Lean & fat	3 oz.	350
Lean only	3 oz.	189
Chuck, pot roast:		
Lean & fat	3 oz.	278
Lean only	3 oz.	182
Fat, separable, cooked	1 oz.	207
Filet mignon (See STEAK, sirloin, lean)		
Flank, braised, 100% lean	3 oz.	167
Ground:		
Regular, raw	½ cup	303
Regular, broiled	3 oz.	243
Lean, broiled	3 oz.	186
Rib:		
Roasted, lean & fat	3 oz.	374
Lean only	3 oz.	205
Round:		
Broiled, lean & fat	3 oz.	222
Lean only	3 oz.	161
Rump:		
Broiled, lean & fat	3 oz.	295
Lean only	3 oz.	177
Steak, club, broiled:		
One 8-oz. steak (weighed without bone before cooking) will give you:		
Lean & fat	5.9 oz.	754
Lean only	3.4 oz.	234
Steak, porterhouse, broiled:		
One 16-oz. steak (weighed with bone before cooking) will give you:		
Lean & fat	10.2 oz.	1339
Lean only	5.9 oz.	372
Steak, ribeye, broiled:		
One 10-oz. steak (weighed without bone before cooking) will give you:		
Lean & fat	7.3 oz.	911
Lean only	3.8 oz.	258
Steak, sirloin, double-bone, broiled:		
One 16-oz. steak (weighed with bone before cooking) will give you:		
Lean & fat	8.9 oz.	1028

Food and Description	Measure or Quantity	Calories
Lean only	5.9 oz.	359
One 12-oz. steak (weighed with bone before cooking) will give you:		
Lean & fat	6.6 oz.	767
Lean only	4.4 oz.	268
Steak, T-bone, broiled:		
One 16-oz. steak (weighed with bone before cooking) will give you:		
Lean & fat	9.8 oz.	1315
Lean only	5.5 oz.	348
BEEF BOUILLON:		
(Herb-Ox):		
Cube	1 cube	6
Packet	1 packet	8
(MBT)	1 packet	14
(Wyler's)	1 cube	6
Low sodium (Featherweight)	1 tsp.	18
BEEF, CHIPPED:		
Cooked, home recipe	½ cup	188
Frozen, creamed:		
(Banquet) creamed, *Entree for One*	4-oz. pkg.	90
(Stouffer's)	5½-oz. serving	231
BEEF DINNER or ENTREE, frozen:		
(Armour):		
Classic Lites, Steak Diane	10-oz. meal	290
Dinner Classics, Burgundy	10½-oz. dinner	330
(Banquet):		
American Favorites, chopped	11-oz. dinner	434
Extra Helping, regular	16-oz. dinner	864
(Blue Star) *Dining Light,* teriyaki	8⅝-oz. dinner	230
(Conagra) *Light & Elegant,* Julienne	8½-oz. entree	260
(Green Giant)		
Baked, boneless ribs in BBQ sauce with corn on the cob	1 meal	390
Twin pouch, burgundy, with rice & carrots	1 meal	280
(Le Menu):		
Chopped sirloin	11½-oz. dinner	390
Yankee pot roast	11-oz. dinner	360
(Morton):		
Regular	11-oz. dinner	272
Light, sliced	11-oz. dinner	260
(Stouffer's) *Lean Cuisine,* Oriental	8⅝-oz. pkg.	280
(Swanson):		
Regular, 4-compartment, chopped sirloin	11½-oz. dinner	350
Hungry Man:		
Chopped	17¼-oz. dinner	600
Sliced	12¼-oz. entree	330

Food and Description	Measure or Quantity	Calories
(Weight Watchers):		
Beefsteak, 2-compartment meal	8¹⁵/₁₆-oz. pkg.	320
Oriental	10-oz. meal	260
BEEF, DRIED, canned:		
(Hormel)	1 oz.	45
(Swift)	1 oz.	47
BEEF GOULASH (Hormel)		
Short Orders	7½-oz. can	230
BEEF, GROUND, SEASONING MIX:		
*(Durkee):		
Regular	1 cup	653
With onion	1 cup	659
(French's) with onion	1⅛-oz. pkg.	100
BEEF HASH, ROAST:		
Canned, *Mary Kitchen* (Hormel):		
Regular	7½-oz. serving	350
Short Orders	7½-oz. can	360
Frozen (Stouffer's)	½ of 11½-oz. pkg.	265
BEEF, PACKAGED		
(Carl Buddig)	1 oz.	38
BEEF, PEPPER ORIENTAL, frozen (La Choy):		
Dinner	12-oz. dinner	250
Entree	12-oz. entree	160
BEEF PIE, frozen:		
(Banquet)	8-oz. pie	449
(Morton)	8-oz. pie	320
(Swanson):		
Regular	8-oz. pie	400
Chunky	10-oz. pie	530
BEEF PUFFS, frozen (Durkee)	1 piece	47
BEEF ROLL (Hormel) Lumberjack	1 oz.	101
BEEF, SHORT RIBS, frozen:		
(Armour) *Dinner Classics,* boneless	10½-oz. dinner	460
(Stouffer's) boneless, with vegetable gravy	½ of 11½-oz. pkg.	350
BEEF SOUP (See SOUP, Beef)		
BEEF SPREAD, ROAST, canned (Underwood)	½ of 4¾-oz. can	140
BEEF STEAK, BREADED (Hormel) frozen	4-oz. serving	370
BEEF STEW:		
Home recipe, made with lean beef chuck	1 cup	218
Canned, regular pack:		
Dinty Moore (Hormel):		
Regular	8-oz. serving	210
Short Orders	7½-oz. can	150
(Libby's)	7½-oz serving	160

11

Food and Description	Measure or Quantity	Calories
Canned, dietetic (Estee)	7½-oz. serving	210
Frozen:		
(Banquet) *Buffet Supper*	2-lb. pkg.	1016
(Green Giant):		
Boil'N Bag	9-oz. entree	180
Twin pouch, with noodles	9-oz. entree	333
(Stouffer's)	10-oz. serving	305
BEEF STEW SEASONING MIX:		
*(Durkee)	1 cup	379
(French's)	1 pkg.	150
BEEF STOCK BASE (French's)	1 tsp.	8
BEEF STROGANOFF, frozen:		
(Armour) *Dinner Classics*	11¼-oz. dinner	370
(Conagra) *Light & Elegant*	9-oz. entree	260
(Le Menu)	9¼ oz. dinner	430
(Stouffer's) with parsley noodles	9¾ oz.	390
***BEEF STROGANOFF SEASONING MIX** (Durkee)	1 cup	820
BEER & ALE:		
Regular:		
Black Horse Ale	8 fl. oz.	108
Black Label (Heilemann)	8 fl. oz.	91
Blatz (Heilemann)	8 fl. oz.	93
Budweiser: Busch Bavarian	8 fl. oz.	100
Michelob	8 fl. oz.	113
Old Milwaukee	8 fl. oz.	95
Pearl Premium	8 fl. oz.	99
Schlitz	8 fl. oz.	100
Stroh Bohemian	8 fl. oz.	84
Light or low carbohydrate:		
Budweiser Light; Natural light	8 fl. oz.	75
Gablinger's	8 fl. oz.	66
Michelob Light	8 fl. oz.	90
Old Milwaukee	8 fl. oz.	80
Pearl Light	8 fl. oz.	60
Schlitz Light	8 fl. oz.	64
Stroh Light	8 fl. oz.	77
BEER, NEAR:		
Goetz Pale	8 fl. oz.	53
(Metbrew)	8 fl. oz.	49
BEET:		
Boiled, whole	2″-dia. beet	16
Boiled, sliced	½ cup	33
Canned, regular pack, solids & liq.:		
(Blue Boy) Harvard	½ cup	100
(Comstock) pickled	½ cup	90
(Del Monte)		
Pickled	4 oz.	77
Sliced	4 oz.	29
(Greenwood)		
Harvard	½ cup	70

Food and Description	Measure or Quantity	Calories
Pickled	½ cup	110
(Stokely-Van Camp) pickled	½ cup	95
Canned, dietetic, solids & liq.:		
(Blue Boy) whole	½ cup	39
(Comstock)	½ cup	30
(Featherweight) sliced	½ cup	45
(Larsen) *Fresh-Lite*	½ cup	40
(S&W) *Nutradiet*, sliced	½ cup	35
BEET PUREE, canned (Larsen)	½ cup	45
BENEDICTINE LIQUEUR (Julius Wile)	1½ fl. oz.	168
BIG H, burger sauce (Hellmann's)	1 T.	71
BIG MAC (See *McDONALD'S*)		
BIG WHEEL (Hostess)	1 piece	170
BISCUIT DOUGH (Pillsbury):		
Baking Powder, *1869 Brand*	1 biscuit	100
Big Country	1 biscuit	95
Big Country, Good 'N Buttery	1 biscuit	100
Buttermilk:		
Regular	1 biscuit	50
Ballard, Oven Ready	1 biscuit	50
Extra Lights	1 biscuit	60
Extra rich, *Hungry Jack*	1 biscuit	65
Fluffy, *Hungry Jack*	1 biscuit	100
Butter Tastin', 1869 Brand	1 biscuit	100
Dinner	1 biscuit	55
Flaky, *Hungry Jack*	1 biscuit	90
Oven Ready, Ballard	1 biscuit	50
BITTERS (Angostura)	1 tsp.	14
BLACKBERRY, fresh, hulled	1 cup	84
BLACKBERRY JELLY:		
Sweetened (Smucker's)	1 T.	53
Dietetic:		
(Diet Delight)	1 T.	12
(Featherweight)	1 T.	16
BLACKBERRY LIQUEUR (Bols)	1 fl. oz.	95
BLACKBERRY PRESERVE OR JAM:		
Sweetened (Smucker's)	1 T.	53
Dietetic:		
(Estee; Louis Sherry)	1 T.	6
(Featherweight)	1 T.	16
(S&W) *Nutradiet*	1 T.	12
BLACKBERRY WINE (Mogen David)	3 fl. oz.	135
BLACK-EYED PEAS:		
Canned:		
(Allen's)	½ cup	100
(Goya)	½ cup	105
Frozen:		
(Birds Eye)	⅓ pkg.	133

13

Food and Description	Measure or Quantity	Calories
(McKenzie; Seabrook Farms)	⅓ pkg.	130
(Southland)	⅕ of 16-oz. pkg.	130
BLINTZE, frozen (King Kold) cheese	2½-oz. piece	132
BLOODY MARY MIX:		
Dry (Bar-Tender's)	1 serving	26
Liquid (Sacramento)	5½-fl. oz. can	39
BLUEBERRY, fresh, whole	½ cup	45
BLUEBERRY PIE (See PIE, Blueberry)		
BLUEBERRY PRESERVE OR JAM:		
Sweetened (Smucker's)	1 T.	53
Dietetic (Louis Sherry)	1 T.	6
BLUEFISH, broiled	3½″ × 3″ × ½″ piece	199
BODY BUDDIES, cereal (General Mills):		
Brown sugar & honey	1 cup	110
Natural fruit flavor	¾ cup	110
BOLOGNA:		
(Eckrich):		
Beef:		
Regular, garlic	1 oz.	90
Thick slice	1½-oz. slice	140
German brand	1-oz. slice	80
Meat, regular	1-oz. slice	90
(Hormel):		
Beef	1-oz. slice	85
Meat	1-oz. slice	90
(Oscar Mayer):		
Beef	.8-oz. slice	73
Beef	1-oz. slice	90
Beef Lebanon	.8-oz. slice	49
Garlic beef	1-oz. slice	89
Meat	1-oz. slice	70
(Swift) *Light & Lean*	1-oz. slice	95
BOLOGNA & CHEESE:		
(Eckrich)	.7-oz. slice	90
(Oscar Mayer)	.8-oz. slice	74
BONITO, canned (Star-Kist):		
Chunk	6½-oz. can	605
Solid	7-oz. can	650
BOO*BERRY, cereal (General Mills)	1 cup	110
BORSCHT, canned:		
Regular:		
(Gold's)	8-oz. serving	72
(Manischewitz)	8-oz. serving	80
(Mother's) old fashioned	8-oz. serving	90
Dietetic or low calorie:		
(Gold's)	8-oz. serving	24
(Manischewitz)	8-oz. serving	20
(Mother's):		
Artificially sweetened	8-oz. serving	29

14

Food and Description	Measure or Quantity	Calories
Unsalted	8-oz. serving	107
(Rokeach):		
Diet	8-oz. serving	15
Unsalted	8-oz. serving	103
BOSCO (See SYRUP)		
BOYSENBERRY JELLY:		
Sweetened (Smucker's)	1 T.	53
Dietetic (S&W) *Nutradiet*, red label	1 T.	12
BRAN:		
Crude	1 oz.	60
Miller's (Elam's)	1 oz.	87
BRAN BREAKFAST CEREAL:		
(Kellogg's):		
All Bran or *Bran Buds*	⅓ cup	70
Cracklin' Oat Bran	½ cup	120
40% bran flakes	¾ cup	90
Raisin	¾ cup	110
(Loma Linda)	1 oz.	90
(Nabisco)	½ cup	70
(Post) 40% bran flakes	⅔ cup	107
(Quaker) *Corn Bran*	⅔ cup	109
(Ralston-Purina):		
Bran Chex	⅔ cup	90
40% bran	¾ cup	100
Raisin	¾ cup	120
BRANDY (See DISTILLED LIQUOR)		
BRANDY, FLAVORED		
(Mr. Boston):		
Apricot	1 fl. oz.	94
Blackberry	1 fl. oz.	92
Cherry	1 fl. oz.	87
Ginger	1 fl. oz.	72
Peach	1 fl. oz.	94
BRAUNSCHWEIGER:		
(Eckrich) chub	1 oz.	70
(Oscar Mayer) chub	1 oz.	96
(Swift) 8-oz. chub	1 oz.	109
BRAZIL NUT:		
Shelled	4 nuts	114
Roasted (Fisher) salted	1 oz.	193
BREAD:		
Boston Brown	3" × ¾" slice	101
Bran'nola (Arnold)	1.3-oz. slice	90
Cinnamon (Pepperidge Farm)	.9-oz. slice	85
Cracked wheat:		
(Pepperidge Farm)	.9-oz. slice	70
(Wonder)	1-oz. slice	70
Crispbread, *Wasa:*		
Rye, lite	.3-oz. slice	30
Sesame	.5-oz. slice	50
Date-nut roll (Dromedary)	1-oz. slice	80

Food and Description	Measure or Quantity	Calories
Flatbread, *Ideal:*		
Bran	.2-oz. slice	19
Extra thin	.1-oz. slice	12
Whole grain	.2-oz. slice	19
French:		
Francisco (Arnold)	1-oz. slice	70
(Wonder)	1-oz. slice	71
Garlic (Arnold)	1-oz. slice	80
Hillbilly	1-oz. slice	70
Hollywood, dark	1-oz. slice	70
Honey bran (Pepperidge Farm)	1-oz. slice	95
Honey wheat berry (Arnold)	1.1-oz. slice	80
Italian (Arnold) *Francisco*	1 slice	70
Multi-grain (Arnold) *Milk & Honey*	1-oz. slice	70
Natural grains (Arnold)	.8-oz. slice	60
Oat (Arnold) *Bran'nola*	1.3-oz. slice	110
Oatmeal (Pepperidge Farm)	.9-oz. slice	70
Pita (see **Sahara**, Thomas')		
Protein (Thomas')	.7-oz. slice	46
Pumpernickel:		
(Arnold)	1-oz. slice	80
(Levy's)	1.1-oz. slice	80
(Pepperidge Farm):		
Regular	1.1-oz. slice	80
Party	.2-oz. slice	17
Raisin:		
(Arnold) tea	.9-oz. slice	70
(Pepperidge Farm)	1 slice	75
(Sun-Maid)	.8-oz. slice	70
Roman Meal	1-oz. slice	70
Rye:		
(Arnold) Jewish	1.1-oz. slice	80
(Levy's) Real	1.1-oz. slice	80
(Pepperidge Farm) family	1.1-oz. slice	85
(Wonder)	1-oz. slice	70
Sahara (Thomas') wheat or white	1-oz. piece	80
Sourdough, *Di Carlo*	1-oz. slice	70
Wheat (see also Cracked Wheat or Whole Wheat):		
(Arnold):		
Bran'nola	1.3-oz. slice	80
Less or *Liteway*	.8-oz. slice	40
Milk & Honey	1-oz. slice	80
Fresh Horizons	1-oz. slice	50
Fresh & Natural	1-oz. slice	70
Home Pride	1-oz. slice	70
(Pepperidge Farm) sandwich	.8-oz. slice	55
(Wonder) family	1-oz. slice	70
Wheatberry, *Home Pride,* honey	1-oz. slice	70
White:		
(Arnold):		
Brick Oven	.8-oz. slice	60

Food and Description	Measure or Quantity	Calories
Country	1.3-oz. slice	100
Less	.8-oz. slice	40
Milk & Honey	1-oz. slice	80
Home Pride	1-oz. slice	72
(Pepperidge Farm):		
Regular	1.2-oz. slice	75
Toasting	1.2-oz. slice	85
(Wonder) regular	1-oz. slice	70
Whole wheat:		
(Arnold) *Stone Ground*	.8-oz. slice	50
(Pepperidge Farm) thin slice	1 slice	65
(Wonder) 100%	1-oz. slice	69
BREAD, CANNED, brown, plain or raisin (B&M)	½″ slice	80
BREAD CRUMBS:		
(Contadina) seasoned	½ cup	211
(Pepperidge Farm)	1 oz.	110
***BREAD DOUGH:**		
Frozen:		
(Pepperidge Farm):		
Country rye or white	1/10 loaf	80
Stone ground wheat	1/10 loaf	75
(Rich's):		
French	1/20 loaf	59
Italian	1/20 loaf	60
Refrigerated (Pillsbury):		
Poppin' Fresh	1/16 loaf	110
***BREAD MIX:**		
Home Hearth:		
French	3/8″ slice	85
Rye or white	3/8″ slice	75
(Pillsbury):		
Banana	1/12 loaf	150
Cherry nut or nut	1/12 loaf	170
BREAD PUDDING, with raisins	½ cup	248
BREAD STICK (Stella D'Oro):		
Plain	1 piece	41
Sesame	1 piece	50
***BREAD STICK DOUGH** (Pillsbury)		
Pipin' Hot	1 piece	100
BREAKFAST BAR (Carnation):		
Almond crunch	1 piece	210
All other varieties	1 piece	200
***BREAKFAST DRINK** (Pillsbury)	1 pouch	290
BREAKFAST SQUARES (General Mills) all flavors	1 bar	190
BROCCOLI:		
Boiled, with stalk	1 stalk (6.3 oz.)	47
Boiled, ½″ pieces	½ cup	20
Frozen:		
(Birds Eye):		
In cheese sauce	1/3 pkg.	87

Food and Description	Measure or Quantity	Calories
Chopped, cuts or florets	⅓ pkg.	31
Spears in butter sauce	⅓ pkg.	58
(Frosty Acres)	3.3 oz.	25
(Green Giant):		
Cuts, polybag	½ cup	18
Spears in butter sauce	3⅓ oz.	40
Spears, mini, *Harvest Fresh*	⅛ pkg.	16
(Seabrook Farms) chopped or spears	⅓ pkg.	30
(Stouffer's) in cheese sauce	½ of 9-oz. pkg.	130
BROTH & SEASONING:		
(George Washington)	1 packet	5
Maggi	1 T.	22
BRUNSWICK STEW, canned		
(Hormel) *Short Orders*	7½-oz. can	220
BRUSSELS SPROUT:		
Boiled	3–4 sprouts	28
Frozen:		
(Birds Eye):		
Regular	⅓ pkg.	6
Baby, with cheese sauce	⅓ pkg.	104
Baby, deluxe	⅓ pkg.	49
(Frosty Acres)	3.3 oz.	35
(Green Giant):		
In butter sauce	½ cup	60
Halves in cheese sauce	½ cup	80
BUCKWHEAT, cracked (Pocono)	1 oz.	104
BUC*WHEATS, cereal (General Mills)	1 oz. (¾ cup)	110
BULGUR, canned, seasoned	4 oz.	206
BURGER KING:		
Apple pie	1 serving	305
Breakfast Croissan'wich:		
Bacon	1 serving	355
Ham	1 serving	335
Sausage	1 serving	538
Cheeseburger:		
Regular	1 serving	304
Double:		
Plain	1 serving	464
bacon	1 serving	510
Condiments:		
Ketchup	1 serving on sandwich	11
Mustard	1 serving on sandwich	2
Pickles	1 serving on sandwich	0
Chicken specialty sandwich:		
Plain	1 serving	492
Condiments:		
Lettuce	1 serving on sandwich	2

Food and Description	Measure or Quantity	Calories
Mayonnaise	1 serving on sandwich	194
Chicken Tenders	1 piece	34
Coffee, regular	1 serving	2
Danish	1 piece	500
Egg platter, scrambled:		
Bacon	1 serving	68
Croissant	1 serving	187
Eggs	1 serving	119
Hash browns	1 serving	162
Sausage	1 serving	234
French fries	1 regular order	227
French toast sticks	1 serving	499
Hamburger:		
Plain	1 burger	262
Condiments:		
Ketchup	1 serving on burger	11
Mustard	1 serving on burger	2
Pickles	1 serving on burger	0
Ham & cheese specialty:		
Plain	1 sandwich	365
Condiments:		
Lettuce	1 serving on sandwich	3
Mayonnaise	1 serving on sandwich	97
Tomato	1 serving on sandwich	6
Milk:		
2% low fat	1 serving	121
Whole	1 serving	157
Onion rings	1 serving	274
Orange juice	1 serving	82
Salad dressing:		
Regular:		
Bleu cheese	1 serving	156
House	1 serving	130
1000 Island	1 serving	117
Dietetic, Italian	1 serving	14
Shakes:		
Chocolate	1 shake	320
Strawberry	1 shake	334
Vanilla	1 shake	321
Soft drink:		
Sweetened:		
Pepsi-Cola	1 regular size	159
7UP	1 regular size	144
Diet *Pepsi*	1 regular size	1
Whaler:		
Plain sandwich	1 sandwich	353

Food and Description	Measure or Quantity	Calories
Condiments:		
Lettuce	1 serving on sandwich	1
Tartar sauce	1 serving on sandwich	134
Whopper:		
Regular:		
Plain	1 sandwich	452
With cheese	1 sandwich	535
Condiments:		
Ketchup	1 serving on sandwich	17
Lettuce	1 serving on sandwich	1
Mayonnaise	1 serving on sandwich	146
Onion	1 serving on sandwich	5
Pickle	1 serving on sandwich	1
Tomato	1 serving on sandwich	6
Junior:		
Plain	1 sandwich	262
With cheese	1 sandwich	305
Condiments:		
Ketchup	1 serving on sandwich	8
Lettuce	1 serving on sandwich	1
Mayonnaise	1 serving on sandwich	48
Pickle	1 serving on sandwich	0
Tomato	1 serving on sandwich	3
Chef's salad	1 serving	180
Garden salad	1 serving	100
Side salad	1 serving	20
Shrimp and pasta	1 serving	170
Croutons	1 packet	30
Dressings:		
Blue cheese	1 packet	310
House	1 packet	260
Reduced-calorie Italian	1 packet	30
Thousand Island	1 packet	235
BURGUNDY WINE:		
(Louis M. Martini)	3 fl. oz.	60
(Paul Masson)	3 fl. oz.	70
(Taylor)	3 fl. oz.	75
BURGUNDY WINE, SPARKLING:		
(Carlo Rossi)	3 fl. oz.	69

Food and Description	Measure or Quantity	Calories
(B&G)	3 fl. oz.	69
(Great Western)	3 fl. oz.	82
(Taylor)	3 fl. oz.	78
BURRITO:		
*Canned (Del Monte)	1 burrito	310
Frozen:		
(Hormel):		
Beef	1 burrito	220
Cheese	1 burrito	250
Hot chili	1 burrito	210
(Swanson) bran & beef	15¼-oz. meal	720
(Van de Kamp's) regular crispy fried	6-oz. serving	365
BURRITO FILLING MIX, canned (Del Monte)	½ cup	110
BUTTER:		
Regular:		
(Breakstone)	1 T.	100
(Meadow Gold)	1 tsp.	35
Whipped (Breakstone)	1 T.	67
BUTTERSCOTCH MORSELS (Nestlé)	1 oz.	150

C

Food and Description	Measure or Quantity	Calories
CABBAGE:		
Boiled, until tender, without salt, drained	1 cup	29
Canned, solids & liq.:		
(Comstock) red	½ cup	60
(Greenwood)	½ cup	60
Frozen (Green Giant) stuffed	½ pkg.	220
CABERNET SAUVIGNON:		
(Louis M. Martini)	3 fl. oz.	63
(Paul Masson)	3 fl. oz.	70
CAFE COMFORT, 55 proof	1 fl. oz.	79
CAKE:		
Regular, non-frozen:		
Plain, home recipe, with butter, with boiled white icing	⅑ of 9″ square	401
Angel food, home recipe	1/12 of 8″ cake	108
Caramel, home recipe, with caramel icing	⅑ of 9″ square	322
Chocolate, home recipe, with chocolate icing, 2-layer	1/12 of 9″ cake	365
Crumb (Hostess)	1¼-oz. cake	130
Fruit:		
Home recipe, dark	1/30 of 8″ loaf	57

Food and Description	Measure or Quantity	Calories
Home recipe, made with butter	1/30 of 8″ loaf	58
(Holland Honey Cake) unsalted	1/14 of cake	80
Pound, home recipe, traditional, made with butter	3½″ × 3½″ slice	123
Raisin date loaf (Holland Honey Cake) low sodium	1/14 of 13-oz. cake	8
Sponge, home recipe	1/12 of 10″ cake	196
White, home recipe, made with butter, without icing, 2-layer	1/9 of 9″ wide, 3″ high cake	353
Yellow, home recipe, made with butter, without icing, 2-layer	1/19 of cake	351
Frozen:		
Banana (Sara Lee)	1/8 of 13¾-oz. cake	175
Butterscotch pecan (Pepperidge Farm) layer	1/10 of 17-oz. cake	160
Carrot:		
(Pepperidge Farm)	1/8 of 11¾-oz. cake	140
(Weight Watchers)	3-oz. serving	180
Cheesecake:		
(Morton) *Great Little Desserts:*		
Cherry	6-oz. cake	460
Cream cheese	6-oz. cake	480
Strawberry	6-oz. cake	470
(Rich's) Viennese	1/14 of 42-oz. cake	230
(Sara Lee):		
Blueberry, *For 2*	½ of 11.3-oz. cake	425
Cream cheese:		
Regular	⅓ of 10-oz. cake	281
Strawberry	⅙ of 19-oz. cake	223
Strawberry, *For 2*	½ of 11.3-oz. cake	420
(Weight Watchers):		
Regular	3.9-oz. serving	200
Strawberry	4-oz. serving	180
Chocolate:		
(Pepperidge Farm):		
Layer, fudge	1/10 of 17-oz. cake	180
Supreme, regular	¼ of 11½-oz. cake	310
(Sara Lee):		
Regular	1/8 of 13¼-oz. cake	199
German	1/8 of 12¼-oz. cake	173
(Weight Watchers) German	2½ oz.	200
Coconut (Pepperidge Farm) layer	1/10 of 17-oz. cake	180
Coffee (Sara Lee):		
Almond	1/8 of 11¾-oz. cake	165
Apple	1/8 of 15-oz. cake	175
Butter, *For 2*	½ of 6½-oz. cake	356
Streusel, butter	1/8 of 11½-oz. cake	164
Crumb (See ROLL OR BUN, Crumb)		

Food and Description	Measure or Quantity	Calories
Devil's food (Pepperidge Farm) layer	⅒ of 17-oz. cake	180
Golden (Pepperidge Farm) layer	⅒ of 17-oz. cake	180
Grand Marnier (Pepperidge Farm)	1½ oz.	160
Lemon coconut (Pepperidge Farm)	¼ of 12¼-oz. cake	280
Orange (Sara Lee)	⅛ of 13¾-oz. cake	179
Pound:		
(Pepperidge Farm) butter	⅒ of 10¾-oz.cake	130
(Sara Lee):		
Regular	⅒ of 10¾-oz. cake	125
Banana nut	⅒ of 11-oz. cake	117
Chocolate	⅒ of 10¾-oz. cake	122
Spice (Weight Watchers)	3-oz. serving	170
Strawberry cream (Pepperidge Farm) Supreme	⅟₁₂ of 12-oz. cake	190
Strawberries'n cream, layer (Sara Lee)	⅛ of 20½-oz. cake	218
Torte (Sara Lee):		
Apples'n cream	⅛ of 21-oz. cake	203
Fudge & nut	⅛ of 15¾-oz. cake	200
Vanilla (Pepperidge Farm) layer	⅒ of 17-oz. cake	180
Walnut, layer (Sara Lee)	⅛ of 18-oz. cake	210
CAKE OR COOKIE ICING		
(Pillsbury) all flavors	1 T.	70
CAKE ICING:		
Butter pecan (Betty Crocker) *Creamy Deluxe*	⅟₁₂ can	170
Caramel, home recipe	4 oz.	408
Cherry (Betty Crocker) *Creamy Deluxe*	⅟₁₂ can	170
Chocolate:		
(Betty Crocker) *Creamy Deluxe:*		
Regular, chip or milk	⅟₁₂ can	170
Sour cream	⅟₁₂ can	160
(Duncan Hines) regular or milk	⅟₁₂ can	163
(Pillsbury) *Frosting Supreme,* fudge, nut or milk	⅟₁₂ can	150
Coconut almond (Pillsbury) *Frosting Supreme*	⅟₁₂ can	150
Cream cheese:		
(Betty Crocker) *Creamy Deluxe*	⅟₁₂ can	170
(Pillsbury) *Frosting Supreme*	⅟₁₂ can	160
Double dutch (Pillsbury) *Frosting Supreme*	⅟₁₂ can	150
Orange (Betty Crocker) *Creamy Deluxe*	⅟₁₂ can	170
Strawberry (Pillsbury) *Frosting Supreme*	⅟₁₂ can	160

Food and Description	Measure or Quantity	Calories
Vanilla:		
(Betty Crocker) *Creamy Deluxe*	⅟₁₂ can	170
(Duncan Hines)	⅟₁₂ can	163
(Pillsbury) *Frosting Supreme,*		
regular or sour cream	⅟₁₂ can	160
White:		
Home recipe, boiled	4 oz.	358
Home recipe, uncooked	4 oz.	426
(Betty Crocker) *Creamy Deluxe*	⅟₁₂ can	160
CAKE ICING MIX:		
Regular:		
Banana (Betty Crocker) *Chiquita,*		
creamy	⅟₁₂ pkg.	170
Butter Brickle (Betty Crocker)		
creamy	⅟₁₂ pkg.	170
Butter pecan (Betty Crocker)		
creamy	⅟₁₂ pkg.	170
Caramel (Pillsbury) *Rich'n Easy*	⅟₁₂ pkg.	140
Cherry (Betty Crocker) creamy	⅟₁₂ pkg.	170
Chocolate:		
Home recipe, fudge	½ cup	586
(Betty Crocker) creamy:		
Fluffy, almond fudge	⅟₁₂ pkg.	180
Fudge, creamy, dark or milk	⅟₁₂ pkg.	170
(Pillsbury) *Rich'n Easy,* fudge or		
milk	⅟₁₂ pkg.	160
Coconut almond (Pillsbury)	⅟₁₂ pkg.	160
Coconut pecan:		
(Betty Crocker) creamy	⅟₁₂ pkg.	140
(Pillsbury)	⅟₁₂ pkg.	150
Cream cheese & nut		
(Betty Crocker) creamy	⅟₁₂ pkg.	150
Lemon:		
(Betty Crocker) *Sunkist,* creamy	⅟₁₂ pkg.	170
(Pillsbury) *Rich'n Easy*	⅟₁₂ pkg.	140
Strawberry (Pillsbury)		
Rich'n Easy	⅟₁₂ pkg.	140
Vanilla (Pillsbury) *Rich'n Easy*	⅟₁₂ pkg.	150
White:		
(Betty Crocker) fluffy	⅟₁₂ pkg.	60
(Betty Crocker) sour cream,		
creamy	⅟₁₂ pkg.	180
(Pillsbury) fluffy	⅟₁₂ pkg.	60
CAKE MEAL (Manischewitz)	½ cup	286
CAKE MIX:		
Regular:		
*Apple (Pillsbury) *Streusel Swirl*	⅟₁₆ of cake	260
Angel Food:		
(Betty Crocker):		
Chocolate or one-step	⅟₁₂ pkg.	140
Traditional	⅟₁₂ pkg.	130
(Duncan Hines)	⅟₁₂ pkg.	124

Food and Description	Measure or Quantity	Calories
*(Pillsbury) raspberry or white	1/12 of cake	140
Applesauce raisin (Betty Crocker)		
Snackin' Cake	1/9 pkg.	180
*Applesauce spice (Pillsbury)	1/12 of cake	250
*Banana:		
(Betty Crocker) *Supermoist*	1/12 of cake	260
(Pillsbury) *Pillsbury Plus*	1/12 of cake	250
*Banana walnut (Betty Crocker)		
Snackin' Cake	1/9 of cake	90
*Boston cream (Pillsbury) *Bundt*	1/16 of cake	270
*Butter (Pillsbury):		
Pillsbury Plus	1/12 of cake	240
Streusel Swirl, rich	1/16 of cake	260
*Butter Brickle (Betty Crocker)		
Supermoist	1/12 of cake	260
*Butter pecan (Betty Crocker)		
Supermoist	1/12 of cake	250
*Carrot (Betty Crocker)		
Supermoist	1/12 of cake	260
*Carrot'n spice (Pillsbury)		
Pillsbury Plus	1/12 of cake	260
*Cheesecake:		
(Jell-O)	1/8 of 8" cake	283
(Royal) No Bake:		
Lite	1/8 of cake	210
Real	1/8 of cake	280
*Cherry chip (Betty Crocker)		
Supermoist	1/12 of cake	180
Chocolate:		
(Betty Crocker):		
*Pudding	1/6 of cake	230
Snackin' Cake:		
Almond	1/9 pkg.	200
Fudge Chip	1/9 pkg.	190
Stir 'N Frost:		
With chocolate frosting	1/6 pkg.	220
Fudge, with vanilla frosting	1/6 pkg.	220
(Duncan Hines):		
Deluxe	1/12 of cake	260
Devil's food	1/12 of cake	280
*Cinnamon (Pillsbury)		
Streusel Swirl	1/16 of cake	260
Coconut pecan (Betty Crocker)		
Snackin' Cake	1/9 pkg.	190
Coffee cake:		
*(Aunt Jemima)	1/8 of cake	170
*(Pillsbury):		
Apple cinnamon	1/8 of cake	240
Cinnamon streusel	1/8 of cake	250
Date nut (Betty Crocker)		
Snackin' Cake	1/9 pkg.	190
*(Pillsbury):		

25

Food and Description	Measure or Quantity	Calories
Bundt:		
Fudge nut crown	1/16 of cake	220
Fudge, tunnel	1/16 of cake	270
Macaroon	1/16 of cake	250
Pillsbury Plus:		
Fudge, dark	1/12 of cake	260
Fudge, marble	1/12 of cake	270
Streusel Swirl, German	1/16 of cake	260
Devil's food:		
*(Betty Crocker) *Supermoist*	1/12 of cake	260
(Duncan Hines) deluxe	1/12 pkg.	190
*(Pillsbury) *Pillsbury Plus*	1/12 of cake	250
Fudge (See Chocolate)		
Golden chocolate chip		
(Betty Crocker) *Snackin' Cake*	1/9 pkg.	190
Lemon:		
(Betty Crocker):		
*Chiffon	1/12 of cake	190
Stir 'N Frost, with lemon		
frosting	1/12 pkg.	230
Supermoist	1/12 cake	260
*(Pillsbury):		
Bundt, tunnel of	1/16 cake	270
Streusel Swirl	1/16 cake	260
*Lemon blueberry (Pillsbury)		
Bundt	1/16 cake	200
Marble:		
*(Betty Crocker) *Supermoist*	1/12 cake	260
*(Pillsbury):		
Bundt, supreme, ring	1/16 cake	250
Streusel Swirl, fudge	1/16 cake	260
*Oats'n brown sugar (Pillsbury)		
Pillsbury Plus	1/12 cake	260
*Pecan brown sugar (Pilisbury)		
Streusel Swirl	1/16 cake	260
*Orange (Betty Crocker)		
Supermoist	1/12 cake	260
Pound:		
*(Betty Crocker) golden	1/12 cake	200
*(Dromedary)	1/2" slice	150
Spice (Betty Crocker):		
Snackin' Cake, raisin	1/9 pkg.	180
Supermoist	1/12 cake	260
Strawberry:		
*(Betty Crocker) *Supermoist*	1/12 cake	260
*(Pillsbury) *Pillsbury Plus*	1/12 cake	260
*Upside down (Betty Crocker)		
pineapple	1/9 cake	270
White:		
*(Betty Crocker):		
Stir 'N Frost, with		
chocolate frosting	1/6 cake	220

Food and Description	Measure or Quantity	Calories
Supermoist	1/12 cake	230
(Duncan Hines) deluxe	1/12 pkg.	188
Yellow:		
*(Betty Crocker) *Supermoist*	1/12 cake	260
(Duncan Hines) deluxe	1/12 pkg.	188
*(Pillsbury) *Pillsbury Plus*	1/12 cake	260
*Dietetic (Estee)	1/10 cake	100
CAMPARI, 45 proof	1 fl. oz.	66
CANDY, REGULAR:		
Almond, Jordan (Banner)	1¼-oz. box	154
Almond Joy (Peter Paul Cadbury)	1.5-oz. bar	220
Apricot Delight (Sahadi)	1 oz.	100
Baby Ruth	2-oz. piece	260
Bar None (Hershey's)	1½ oz.	240
Bonkers! any flavor	1 piece	20
Breath Savers (Life Savers)	1 piece	8
Butterfinger	2-oz. bar	260
Butternut (Hollywood Brands)	2¼-oz. bar	310
Caramel:		
Caramel Flipper (Wayne)	1 oz.	128
Caramel Nip (Pearson)	1 piece	30
Charleston Chew	2-oz. piece	240
Cherry, chocolate-covered		
(Welch's) dark	1 piece	90
Chocolate bar:		
Brazil nut (Cadbury's)	2 oz.	310
Caramello (Cadbury's)	2 oz.	280
Crunch (Nestlé)	1 1/16-oz. bar	160
Hazelnut (Cadbury's)	2 oz.	310
Milk:		
(Cadbury's)	2 oz.	300
(Hershey's)	1.65-oz. bar	250
(Nestlé)	.35-oz. bar	53
(Nestlé)	1 1/16-oz. bar	159
Special Dark (Hershey's)	1.45-oz. bar	220
Chocolate bar with almonds:		
(Cadbury's)	2 oz.	310
(Hershey's) milk	1.55-oz. bar	250
(Nestlé)	1 oz.	160
Chocolate Parfait (Pearson)	1 piece	30
Chocolate, Petite (Andes)	1 piece	26
Chuckles	1 oz.	92
Clark Bar	1.5-oz. bar	201
Coffee Nip (Pearson)	1 piece	30
Coffioca Parfait (Pearson)	1 piece	30
Creme de Menthe (Andes)	1 piece	25
Crispy Bar (Clark)	1¼-oz. bar	187
Crows (Mason)	1 piece	11
Dutch Treat Bar (Clark)	1 1/16-oz. bar	160
Eggs (Peter Paul Cadbury) creme	1 oz.	136
5th Avenue (Hershey's)	1.93-oz. bar	270

Food and Description	Measure or Quantity	Calories
Fudge (Nabisco) bar	1 piece	85
Good Stuff (Nab)	1.8-oz. piece	250
Halvah (Sahadi) original and marble	1 oz.	150
Hard (Jolly Rancher):		
All flavors except butterscotch	1 piece	23
Butterscotch	1 piece	25
Hollywood	1½-oz. bar	185
Jelly bean, *Chuckles*	.5 oz.	55
Jelly rings, *Chuckles*	1 piece	37
Jujubes, Chuckles	.5 oz.	55
Ju Jus:		
Assorted	1 piece	7
Coins or raspberries	1 piece	15
Kisses (Hershey's)	1 piece	24
Kit Kat	1.6-oz. bar	250
Krackel Bar	.35-oz. bar	52
Krackel Bar	1.6-oz. bar	250
Licorice:		
(Switzer) bars, bites or stix:		
Black	1 oz.	94
Cherry or strawberry	1 oz.	98
Chocolate	1 oz.	97
Twist:		
Black (American Licorice Co.)	1 piece	27
Black (Curtiss)	1 piece	27
Red (American Licorice Co.)	1 piece	33
Life Savers	1 piece	10
Lollipops (Life Savers)	1 pop	45
Mallo Cup (Boyer)	9/16-oz. piece	54
Malted milk balls (Brach's)	1 piece	9
Mars Bar (M&M/Mars)	1.7-oz. bar	240
Marshmallow (Campfire)	1 oz.	111
Mary Jane (Miller):		
Small size	1.4 oz.	19
Large size	1½-oz. bar	110
Milk Duds (Clark)	¾-oz. box	89
Milk Shake (Hollywood Brands)	2.4-oz. bar	300
Milky Way (M&M/Mars)	2.24-oz. bar	290
Mint or peppermint:		
After dinner (Richardson):		
Jelly center	1 oz.	104
Regular	1 oz.	109
Chocolate covered (Richardson)	1 oz.	106
Junior mint pattie (Nabisco)	1 piece	10
Mint Parfait (Andes)	1 piece	27
Peppermint Pattie (Nabisco)	1 piece	55
York, pattie (Peter Paul Cadbury)	1¼-oz. serving	160
M & M's:		
Peanut	1.83-oz. pkg.	270
Plain	1.69-oz. pkg.	240
Mounds (Peter Paul Cadbury)	1.65-oz. serving	230

Food and Description	Measure or Quantity	Calories
Mr. Goodbar (Hershey's)	1.8-oz. bar	300
Munch Bar (M&M/Mars)	1.42-oz. bar	220
My Buddy (Tom's)	1.8-oz. piece	250
Naturally Nut & Fruit Bar (Planters) almond/apricot	1 oz.	140
$100,000 Bar (Nestlé)	1¼-oz. bar	175
Orange slices, *Chuckles*	1 oz.	110
Park Avenue (Tom's)	1.8-oz. bar	230
Payday (Hollywood Brands) regular	1.9-oz. bar	250
Peanut bar (Planters)	1.6 oz.	240
Peanut, chocolate-covered:		
(Curtiss)	1 piece	5
(Nabisco)	1 piece	11
Peanut butter cup:		
(Boyer)	1.5-oz. pkg.	148
(Reese's)	.9-oz. cup	140
Peanut Butter Pals (Tom's)	1.3-oz. serving	200
Peanut crunch bar (Sahadi)	¾-oz. bar	110
Peanut Parfait (Andes)	1 piece	28
Peanut Plank (Tom's)	1.7-oz. piece	230
Peanut Roll (Tom's)	1.75-oz. piece	230
Powerhouse (Peter Paul Cadbury)	2 oz.	260
Raisin, chocolate-covered:		
(Nabisco)	1 piece	5
Raisinets (BB)	1 oz.	140
Reese's Pieces (Hershey's)	1.95-oz. pkg.	270
Reggie Bar	2-oz. bar	290
Rolo (Hershey's)	1 piece	30
Royals, mint chocolate (M&M/Mars)	1.52-oz. pkg.	212
Sesame Crunch (Sahadi)	¾-oz. bar	110
Skor (Hershey's)	1.4-oz. bar	220
Snickers	2-oz. bar	290
Spearmint leaves, *Chuckles*	1 oz.	110
Starburst (M&M/Mars)	1-oz. serving	120
Sugar Babies (Nabisco)	1.6-oz. pkg.	180
Sugar Daddy (Nabisco) caramel sucker	1.4-oz. pop	150
Sugar Mama (Nabisco)	¾-oz. pop	90
Summit bar (M&M/Mars)	1 bar	115
Taffy:		
Salt water (Brach's)	1 piece	31
Turkish (Bonomo)	1 oz.	108
3 Musketeers	.8-oz. bar	99
3 Musketeers	2.1-oz. bar	260
Ting-A-Ling (Andes)	1 piece	24
Tootsie Roll:		
Chocolate	.23-oz. midgee	26
Chocolate	1/16-oz. bar	72
Chocolate	1-oz. bar	115
Flavored	.6-oz. square	19

Food and Description	Measure or Quantity	Calories
Pop, all flavors	.49-oz. pop	55
Pop drop, all flavors	4.7-gram piece	19
Twix Cookie bar (M&M/Mars)	1¾-oz. serving	246
Peanut butter cookie bar (M&M/Mars)	1¾-oz. serving	261
Twizzlers	1 oz.	100
Whatchamacallit (Hershey's)	1.8-oz. bar	260
Wispa (Peter Paul Cadbury)	1 oz.	150
World Series Bar	1 oz.	128
Y & S Bites	1 oz.	100
Zagnut Bar (Clark)	.7-oz. bar	85
Zero (Hollywood Brands)	2-oz. bar	210
CANDY, DIETETIC:		
Carob bar, *Joan's Natural:*		
Coconut	3-oz. bar	516
Fruit & nut	3-oz. bar	559
Honey bran	3-oz. bar	487
Peanut	3-oz. bar	521
Chocolate or chocolate-flavored bar:		
(Estee):		
Coconut, fruit & nut or milk	.2-oz. square	30
Crunch	.2-oz. square	22
(Louis Sherry) coffee or orange flavored	.2-oz. square	22
Estee-ets, with peanuts (Estee)	1 piece	7
Gum drops (Estee) any flavor	1 piece	3
Gummy Bears (Estee)	1 piece	5
Hard candy:		
(Estee) assorted fruit	1 piece	11
(Louis Sherry)	1 piece	12
Mint:		
(Estee)	1 piece	4
(Sunkist):		
Mini mint	1 piece	1
Roll mint	1 piece	4
Peanut butter cup (Estee)	1 cup	45
Raisins, chocolate-covered (Estee)	1 piece	5
CANNELLONI, frozen:		
(Blue Star) *Dining Light*, cheese	9-oz. dinner	261
(Celentano)	12-oz. pkg.	380
(Stouffer's) beef & pork with mornay sauce	9⅝-oz. pkg.	240
(Weight Watchers) one-compartment	13-oz. meal	450
CANTALOUPE, cubed	½ cup (3 oz.)	24
CAPERS (Crosse & Blackwell)	1 tsp.	2
CAP'N CRUNCH, cereal (Quaker):		
Regular	¾ cup	121
Crunchberry	¾ cup	120
Peanut butter	¾ cup	127
CAPOCOLLO (Hormel)	1 oz.	80

Food and Description	Measure or Quantity	Calories
CARAWAY SEED (French's)	1 tsp.	8
CARNATION DO-IT-YOURSELF DIET PLAN	2 scoops	110
CARNATION INSTANT BREAKFAST:		
Bar:		
Chocolate chip	1 bar	200
Peanut butter crunch	1 bar	180
Packets, all flavors	1 packet	130
CARROT:		
Raw	5½″ × 1″ piece	21
Boiled, slices	½ cup	24
Canned, regular pack, solids & liq.:		
(Comstock)	½ cup	35
(Del Monte) sliced or whole	½ cup	30
(Libby's)	½ cup	20
Canned, dietetic pack, solids & liq., (S&W) *Nutradiet*, green label	½ cup	30
Frozen:		
(Birds Eye) whole, baby deluxe	⅓ pkg.	84
(Frosty Acres)	3.3 oz.	40
(Green Giant) cuts, in butter sauce	½ cup	80
(Seabrook Farms)	⅓ pkg.	39
CARROT PUREE (Larsen)	½ cup	35
CASABA MELON	1-lb. melon	61
CASHEW NUT:		
(Fisher):		
Dry roasted	1 oz.	156
Oil roasted	1 oz.	159
(Planters):		
Dry roasted	1 oz.	160
Oil roasted	1 oz.	170
CATFISH, frozen (Mrs. Paul's) breaded-fried, fingers	4 oz.	250
CATSUP:		
Regular:		
(Del Monte)	1 T.	17
(Heinz)	1 T.	18
(Smucker's)	1 T.	21
Dietetic or low calorie:		
(Del Monte) No Salt Added	1 T.	15
(Featherweight)	1 T.	6
(Heinz) lite	1 T.	8
CAULIFLOWER:		
Raw or boiled buds	½ cup	14
Frozen:		
(Birds Eye) regular or florets, deluxe	⅓ pkg.	28
(Frosty Acres)	3.3 oz.	25
(Green Giant) in cheese sauce	½ cup	60
CAVATELLI, frozen (Celentano)	⅕ of 16-oz. pkg.	270

Food and Description	Measure or Quantity	Calories
CAVIAR:		
Pressed	1 oz.	90
Whole eggs	1 T.	42
CELERY:		
1 large outer stalk	8″ × 1½″ at root end	7
Diced or cut	½ cup	9
Salt (French's)	1 tsp.	12
Seed (French's)	1 tsp.	11
CERTS	1 piece	6
CERVELAT (Hormel) Viking	1-oz. serving	90
CHABLIS WINE:		
(Almaden) light	3 fl. oz.	42
(Carlo Rossi)	3 fl. oz.	66
(Gallo) white or pink	3 fl. oz.	60
(Louis M. Martini)	3 fl. oz.	59
(Paul Masson):		
Regular	3 fl. oz.	71
Light	3 fl. oz.	45
CHAMPAGNE:		
(Bollinger)	3 fl. oz.	72
(Great Western):		
Regular	3 fl. oz.	71
Brut	3 fl. oz.	74
Pink	3 fl. oz.	81
(Taylor) dry	3 fl. oz.	78
CHARDONNAY WINE		
(Louis M. Martini)	3 fl. oz.	61
CHARLOTTE RUSSE,		
homemade recipe	4 oz.	324
CHEERIOS, cereal, regular or		
honey & nut	1 oz.	110
CHEESE:		
American or cheddar:		
Cube, natural	1″ cube	68
(Borden)	1 oz.	110
(Dorman's) *Chedda-De Lite*	1 oz.	90
(Kraft):		
American Singles	1 oz.	90
Cheddar	1 oz.	110
Old English	1 oz.	110
Laughing Cow, natural	1 oz.	110
(Sargento):		
Midget, regular or sharp	1 oz.	114
Shredded, non-dairy	1 oz.	90
Wispride	1 oz.	115
Blue:		
(Frigo)	1 oz.	100
(Kraft)	1 oz.	100
(Sargento) cold pack or crumbled	1 oz.	100
Bonbino, *Laughing Cow,* natural	1 oz.	103
Brick (Sargento)	1 oz.	105
Brie (Sargento) *Danish Danko*	1 oz.	80

Food and Description	Measure or Quantity	Calories
Burgercheese (Sargento)		
Danish Danko	1 oz.	106
Camembert (Sargento)		
Danish Danko	1 oz.	88
Colby:		
(Featherweight) low sodium	1 oz.	100
(Kraft)	1 oz.	110
(Pauly) low sodium	1 oz.	115
(Sargento) shredded or sliced	1 oz.	112
Cottage:		
Unflavored:		
(Bison):		
Regular	1 oz.	29
Dietetic	1 oz.	22
(Breakstone's) smooth &		
creamy	1 oz.	27
(Dairylea)	1 oz.	30
(Friendship)	1 oz.	30
(Light n' Lively)	1 oz.	20
(Sealtest)	1 oz.	30
Flavored (Friendship)		
Dutch apple	1 oz.	31
Cream, plain, unwhipped:		
(Frigo)	1 oz.	100
(Kraft) *Philadelphia Brand*:		
Regular	1 oz.	100
Light	1 oz.	60
Edam:		
(House of Gold)	1 oz.	100
(Kaukauna)	1 oz.	100
(Kraft)	1 oz.	90
Laughing Cow	1 oz.	100
Farmers:		
Dutch Garden Brand	1 oz.	100
(Kaukauna)	1 oz.	100
(Sargento)	1 oz.	72
Wispride	1 oz.	100
Feta (Sargento) cups	1 oz.	76
Gjetost (Sargento) Norwegian	1 oz.	118
Gouda:		
(Kaukauna)	1 oz.	100
Laughing Cow	1 oz.	110
(Sargento) baby, caraway		
or smoked	1 oz.	101
Wispride	1 oz.	100
Gruyère, *Swiss Knight*	1 oz.	100
Havarti (Sargento):		
Creamy	1 oz.	90
Creamy, 60% mild	1 oz.	117
Hoop (Friendship) natural	1 oz.	21
Hot pepper (Sargento)	1 oz.	112
Jarlsberg (Sargento) Norwegian	1 oz.	100

Food and Description	Measure or Quantity	Calories
Kettle Moraine (Sargento)	1 oz.	100
Limburger (Sargento) natural	1 oz.	93
Monterey Jack:		
(Frigo)	1 oz.	100
(Kaukauna)	1 oz.	110
(Sargento) midget, Longhorn, shredded or sliced	1 oz.	106
Mozzarella:		
(Fisher) part skim milk	1 oz.	90
(Kraft)	1 oz.	80
(Polly-O) Lite	1 oz.	70
(Sargento):		
Bar, rounds, shredded regular or with spices, sliced for pizzas or square	1 oz.	79
Whole milk	1 oz.	100
Muenster:		
(Dorman's)	1 oz.	110
(Kaukauna)	1 oz.	110
(Sargento) red rind	1 oz.	104
Wispride	1 oz.	100
Nibblin Curds (Sargento)	1 oz.	114
Parmesan:		
(Frigo):		
Grated	1 T.	23
Whole	1 oz.	110
(Sargento):		
Grated	1 T.	27
Wedge	1 oz.	110
Pizza (Sargento) shredded or sliced	1 oz.	90
Pot (Sargento) regular, French onion or garlic	1 oz.	30
Provolone:		
(Frigo)	1 oz.	90
Laughing Cow:		
Cube	⅙ oz.	12
Wedge	¾ oz.	55
(Sargento) sliced	1 oz.	100
Ricotta:		
(Frigo) part skim milk	1 oz.	43
(Sargento):		
Part skim milk	1 oz.	39
Whole milk	1 oz.	49
Romano (Sargento) wedge	1 oz.	110
Roquefort, natural	1 oz.	104
Samsoe (Sargento) Danish	1 oz.	79
Scamorze (Frigo)	1 oz.	79
Semisoft, *Laughing Cow:*		
Babybel	1 oz.	90
Bonbel	1 oz.	100
Slim Jack (Dorman's)	1 oz.	90
Stirred curd (Frigo)	1 oz.	110

Food and Description	Measure or Quantity	Calories
String (Sargento)	1 oz.	90
Swiss:		
(Dorman's)	1 oz.	100
(Fisher) natural	1 oz.	100
(Frigo) domestic	1 oz.	100
(Sargento) domestic or Finland, sliced	1 oz.	107
Taco (Sargento) shredded	1 oz.	105
Washed curd (Frigo)	1 oz.	110
CHEESE FONDUE, *Swiss Knight*	1 oz.	110
CHEESE FOOD:		
American or cheddar:		
(Borden) *Lite Line*	1 oz.	50
(Fisher) *Ched-O-Mate* or *Sandwich-Mate*	1 oz.	90
(Weight Watchers) colored or white	1-oz. slice	50
Wispride:		
Regular	1 oz.	100
& port wine	1 oz.	100
Cheez-ola (Fisher)	1 oz.	90
Chef's Delight (Fisher)	1 oz.	70
Count Down (Pauly)	1 oz.	40
Cracker snack (Sargento)	1 oz.	90
Garlic & herbs, *Wispride*	1 oz.	90
Jalapeño (Borden) *Lite Line*	1 oz.	50
Loaf, *Count Down* (Pauly)	1 oz.	100
Low sodium (Borden) *Lite Line*	1 oz.	70
Monterey Jack (Borden) *Lite Line*	1 oz.	50
Mun-chee (Pauly)	1 oz.	100
Pimiento (Pauly)	.8-oz. slice	73
Pizza-Mate (Fisher)	1 oz.	90
Swiss:		
(Borden) *Lite Line*	1 oz.	50
(Kraft) reduced fat	1 oz.	90
CHEESE PUFFS, frozen (Durkee)	1 piece	59
CHEESE SPREAD:		
American or cheddar:		
(Fisher)	1 oz.	80
Laughing Cow	1 oz.	72
(Nabisco) *Easy Cheese*	1 tsp.	16
Blue, *Laughing Cow*	1 oz.	72
Cheese'n Bacon (Nabisco) *Easy Cheese*	1 tsp.	16
Gruyère, *Laughing Cow, La Vache Que Rit*, reduced calorie	1 oz.	46
Provolone, *Laughing Cow*	1 oz.	72
Sharp (Pauly)	.8 oz.	77
Swiss, process (Pauly)	.8 oz.	76
Velveeta (Kraft)	1 oz.	80
CHEESE STRAW, frozen (Durkee)	1 piece	29
CHENIN BLANC WINE (Louis M. Martini)	3 fl. oz.	60

Food and Description	Measure or Quantity	Calories
CHERRY, sweet:		
Fresh, with stems	½ cup	41
Canned, regular pack (Del Monte)		
dark, solids & liq.	½ cup	50
Canned, dietetic, solids & liq.:		
(Diet Delight) with pits,		
water pack	½ cup	70
(Featherweight) dark, water pack	½ cup	60
(Thank You Brand)	½ cup	61
CHERRY, CANDIED	1 oz.	96
CHERRY DRINK:		
Canned:		
(Hi-C)	6 fl. oz.	93
(Lincoln) cherry berry	6 fl. oz.	100
*Mix (Hi-C)	6 fl. oz.	72
CHERRY HEERING		
(Hiram Walker)	1 fl. oz.	80
CHERRY JELLY:		
Sweetened (Smucker's)	1 T.	53
Dietetic:		
(Dia-Mel)	1 T.	6
(Featherweight)	1 T.	16
CHERRY LIQUEUR (DeKuyper)	1 fl. oz.	75
CHERRY PRESERVES OR JAM:		
Sweetened (Smucker's)	1 T.	53
Dietetic (Estee)	1 T.	6
CHESTNUT, fresh, in shell	¼ lb.	220
CHEWING GUM:		
Sweetened:		
Bazooka, bubble	1 slice	18
Beechies	1 piece	6
Beech Nut; Beeman's Big Red;		
Black Jack; Clove; Doublemint;		
Freedent; Juicy Fruit,		
Spearmint (Wrigley's);		
Teaberry	1 stick	10
Bubble Yum	1 piece	25
Extra (Wrigley's)	1 piece	8
Fruit Stripe, regular	1 piece	9
Dentyne	1 piece	4
Hubba Bubba (Wrigley's)	1 piece	23
Dietetic:		
Bubble Yum	1 piece	20
Care Free, regular	1 piece	8
(Clark; *Care*Free*)	1 piece	7
(Estee) bubble or regular	1 piece	5
(Featherweight) bubble or regular	1 piece	4
Orbit (Wrigley's)	1 piece	8
CHEX, cereal (Ralston Purina):		
Corn	1 cup	110
Rice	1 cup	110
Wheat	⅔ cup	110
Wheat & raisins	¾ cup	130

Food and Description	Measure or Quantity	Calories
CHIANTI WINE:		
(Italian Swiss Colony)	3 fl. oz.	83
(Louis M. Martini)	3 fl. oz.	90
CHICKEN:		
Broiler, cooked, meat only	3 oz.	116
Fryer, fried, meat & skin	3 oz.	212
Fryer, fried, meat only	3 oz.	178
Fryer, fried, 2½-lb. chicken (weighed with bone before cooking) will give you:		
Back	1 back	139
Breast	½ breast	160
Leg or drumstick	1 leg	87
Neck	1 neck	127
Rib	1 rib	41
Thigh	1 thigh	122
Wing	1 wing	82
Fried skin	1 oz.	119
Hen & cock:		
Stewed, dark meat only	3 oz.	176
Stewed, diced	½ cup	139
Stewed, light meat only	3 oz.	153
Stewed, meat & skin	3 oz.	269
Roaster, roasted, dark or light meat, without skin	3 oz.	156
CHICKEN À LA KING:		
Home recipe	1 cup	468
Canned (Swanson)	½ of 10½-oz. can	180
Frozen:		
(Banquet) *Cookin' Bag*	4-oz. pkg.	110
(Blue Star) *Dining Lite,* with rice	9½-oz. entree	290
(Green Giant) twin pouch, with biscuits	9-oz. entree	370
(Le Menu)	10¼-oz. dinner	320
(Stouffer's) with rice	9½-oz. pkg.	330
(Weight Watchers)	9-oz. pkg.	230
CHICKEN, BONED, canned:		
Regular:		
(Hormel) chunk, breast	6¾-oz. serving	350
(Swanson) chunk:		
Mixin' chicken	2½ oz.	130
White	2½ oz.	90
Low sodium (Featherweight)	2½ oz.	154
CHICKEN BOUILLON:		
(Herb-Ox):		
Cube	1 cube	6
Packet	1 packet	12
(Wyler's)	1 cube	8
Low sodium (Featherweight)	1 tsp.	18
CHICKEN, CREAMED, frozen (Stouffer's)	6½ oz.	300

Food and Description	Measure or Quantity	Calories
CHICKEN DINNER OR ENTREE:		
Canned (Swanson) & dumplings	7½ oz.	220
Frozen:		
(Armour):		
Classic Lites:		
Burgundy	11¼-oz. dinner	230
Sweet & sour	11-oz. dinner	250
Dinner Classics:		
Fricassee	11¾-oz. dinner	340
Milan	11½-oz. dinner	350
(Banquet):		
American Favorites	11-oz. dinner	359
Family Entrees	32-oz. pkg.	1720
(Blue Star) *Dining Lite,* glazed	8½-oz. dinner	243
(Celentano):		
Parmigiana	9-oz. meal	310
Primavera	11½-oz. pkg.	270
(Conagra) *Light & Elegant:*		
Cheese	8¾-oz. entree	293
Parmigiana	8-oz. entree	260
(Green Giant):		
Baked:		
In BBQ sauce with corn on the cob	1 meal	350
Stir fry and garden vegetables	10-oz. entree	250
(Le Menu) sweet & sour	11¼-oz. dinner	450
(Morton):		
Regular:		
Boneless	11-oz. dinner	329
Fried	11-oz. pkg.	431
Light, boneless	11-oz. dinner	250
(Stouffer's):		
Regular:		
Cacciatore, with spaghetti	11¼-oz. meal	313
Divan	8½-oz. serving	336
Lean Cuisine:		
Glazed with vegetable rice	8½-oz. serving	270
& vegetables with vermicelli	12¾-oz. serving	260
(Swanson):		
Regular:		
& dumplings	7½-oz. meal	220
Fried, 4-compartment:		
Barbecue flavor	9¼-oz. dinner	560
Dark meat	10¼-oz. dinner	610
Hungry Man:		
Boneless	17½-oz. dinner	670
Parmigiana	20-oz. dinner	810
(Tyson):		
A l'orange	8¼-oz. meal	300
Français	8¾-oz. meal	350
Parmigiana	11¾-oz. meal	450
(Weight Watchers):		

38

Food and Description	Measure or Quantity	Calories
Cacciatore	10-oz. serving	290
Imperial	9¼-oz. meal	240
Parmigiana	8-oz. serving	290
CHICKEN, FRIED, frozen:		
(Banquet) assorted	2-lb. pkg.	1625
(Swanson) *Plump & Juicy:*		
Assorted	3¼-oz. serving	270
Breast portions	4½-oz. serving	350
Nibbles	3¼-oz. serving	300
Take-out style	3¼-oz. serving	270
CHICKEN & NOODLES, frozen:		
(Green Giant) twin pouch, with vegetables	9-oz. pkg.	365
(Stouffer's):		
Escalloped	5¾-oz. serving	252
Paprikash	10½-oz. serving	391
CHICKEN NUGGETS, frozen		
(Banquet) regular	12-oz. pkg.	932
CHICKEN, PACKAGED:		
(Carl Buddig) smoked	1 oz.	50
(Louis Rich) breast, oven roasted	1-oz. slice	40
CHICKEN PATTY, frozen (Banquet)	12-oz. pkg.	900
CHICKEN PIE, frozen:		
(Banquet) regular	8-oz. pie	450
(Stouffer's)	10-oz. pie	493
(Swanson) regular	8-oz. pie	420
CHICKEN PUFF, frozen (Durkee)	½-oz. piece	49
CHICKEN SALAD (Carnation)	¼ of 7½-oz. can	94
CHICKEN SOUP (See SOUP, Chicken)		
CHICKEN SPREAD:		
(Hormel) regular	1 oz.	60
(Underwood) chunky	½ of 4¾-oz. can	63
CHICKEN STEW, canned:		
Regular:		
(Libby's) with dumplings	8 oz.	194
(Swanson)	7⅜ oz.	170
Dietetic (Dia-Mel)	8-oz. serving	150
CHICKEN STOCK BASE (French's)	1 tsp.	8
CHICK-FIL-A:		
Sandwich	5.4-oz. serving	404
Soup, hearty, breast of chicken:		
Small	8⅕ oz.	131
Large	14.3 oz.	230
CHICK'N QUICK, frozen (Tyson):		
Breast fillet	3 oz.	190
Breast pattie	3 oz.	240
Chick'N Cheddar	3 oz.	260
Cordon bleu	5 oz.	310
Kiev	5 oz.	430
CHICK PEA OR GARBANZO, canned, solids & liq.		
(Allen's; Goya)	½ cup	110

Food and Description	Measure or Quantity	Calories
CHILI OR CHILI CON CARNE:		
Canned, regular pack:		
Beans only:		
(Comstock)	½ cup	140
(Hormel)	5 oz.	130
(Van Camp) Mexican style	1 cup	250
With beans:		
(Hormel) regular or hot	7½-oz. serving	310
(Libby's)	7½-oz. serving	270
(*Old El Paso*)	1 cup	349
(Swanson)	7¾-oz. serving	310
Without beans:		
(Hormel) regular or hot	7½-oz. serving	370
(Libby's)	7½ oz.	390
Canned, dietetic pack:		
(Estee) with beans	8-oz. serving	390
(Featherweight) with beans	7½ oz.	270
Frozen, with beans (Stouffer's)	8¾-oz. pkg.	270
CHILI SAUCE:		
(Del Monte)	¼ cup (2 oz.)	70
(Heinz)	1 T.	17
(Ortega) green, medium	1 oz.	7
(Featherweight) Dietetic	1 T.	8
CHILI SEASONING MIX:		
*(Durkee)	1 cup	465
(French's) *Chili-O*, plain	1¾-oz. pkg.	150
(McCormick)	1.2-oz. pkg.	106
CHOCO-DILE (Hostess)	2-oz. piece	235
CHOCOLATE, BAKING:		
(Baker's):		
Bitter or unsweetened	1 oz.	180
Semi-sweet, chips	½ cup	207
Sweetened, *German's*	1 oz.	158
(Hershey's):		
Bitter or unsweetened	1 oz.	190
Sweetened:		
Dark chips, regular or mini	1 oz.	151
Milk, chips	1 oz.	150
Semi-sweet, chips	1 oz.	147
(Nestlé):		
Bitter or unsweetened, *Choco-bake*	1-oz. packet	180
Sweet or semi-sweet, morsels	1 oz.	150
CHOCOLATE ICE CREAM		
(See ICE CREAM, Chocolate)		
CHOCOLATE SYRUP		
(See SYRUP, Chocolate)		
CHOP SUEY, frozen (Stouffer's) beef with rice	12-oz. pkg.	355
***CHOP SUEY SEASONING MIX** (Durkee)	1¾ cups	557
CHOWDER (See SOUP, Chowder)		

Food and Description	Measure or Quantity	Calories
CHOW MEIN:		
Canned:		
(Chun King) Divider-Pak:		
Beef	¼ of pkg.	91
Chicken	½ of 24-oz pkg.	110
Shrimp	¼ of pkg.	91
(Hormel) Pork, *Short Orders*	7½-oz. can	140
(La Choy):		
Regular:		
Beef	1 cup	72
Chicken	½ of 1-lb. can	68
Shrimp	1 cup	61
*Bi-pack:		
Beef or vegetable	¾ cup	60
Beef pepper oriental, chicken or shrimp	¾ cup	70
Pork	¾ cup	90
Frozen:		
(Armour) *Classic Lites*	10½-oz. meal	220
(Blue Star) *Dining Light*, chicken & rice	11¼-oz. dinner	233
(La Choy):		
Chicken	11-oz. dinner	356
Shrimp	11-oz. dinner	323
(Morton) chicken, light	8-oz. entree	210
(Stouffer's) *Lean Cuisine*, with rice	11¼-oz. serving	240
CHOW MEIN SEASONING MIX (Kikkoman)	1⅛-oz. pkg.	98
CHUTNEY (Major Grey's)	1 T.	53
CINNAMON, GROUND (French's)	1 tsp.	6
CITRUS BERRY BLEND, mix, dietetic (Sunkist)	8 fl. oz.	6
CITRUS COOLER DRINK, canned (Hi-C)	6 fl. oz.	93
CLAM:		
Raw, all kinds, meat only	1 cup (8 oz.)	186
Raw, soft, meat & liq.	1 lb. (weighed in shell)	142
Canned (Doxsee):		
Chopped, minced or whole:		
Solids & liquid	½ cup	97
Drained solids	½ cup	58
Canned (Gorton's) minced, meat only	1 can	140
Frozen:		
(Gorton's) fried strips, crunchy	1 package	480
(Howard Johnson's)	5-oz. pkg.	395
(Mrs. Paul's) fried, light	2½-oz. serving	230
CLAMATO COCKTAIL (Mott's)	6 fl. oz.	80
CLAM JUICE (Snow)	½ cup	15

Food and Description	Measure or Quantity	Calories
CLARET WINE:		
(Gold Seal)	3 fl. oz.	82
(Taylor) 12.5% alcohol	3 fl. oz.	72
CLORETS, gum or mint	1 piece	6
COCKTAIL (see individual listings such as **DAIQUIRI, PIÑA COLADA,** etc.)		
COCOA:		
Dry, unsweetened:		
(Hershey's)	1 T.	30
(Sultana)	1 T.	30
Mix, regular:		
(Alba '66) instant, all flavors	1 envelope	60
(Carnation) all flavors	1-oz. pkg.	110
(Hershey's) instant	3 T.	81
(Ovaltine) hot 'n rich	1 oz.	120
Swiss Miss, regular or with mini marshmallows	6 fl. oz.	110
Mix, dietetic:		
(Carnation):		
70 Calorie	¾-oz. packet	70
*Sugar free	6 fl. oz.	50
*(Featherweight)	6 fl. oz.	50
Swiss Miss, instant, lite	3 T.	70
COCOA KRISPIES, cereal		
(Kellogg's)	¾ cup	110
COCOA PUFFS, cereal		
(General Mills)	1 oz.	110
COCONUT:		
Fresh, meat only	2″ × 2″ × ½″ piece	156
Grated or shredded, loosely packed	½ cup	225
Dried:		
(Baker's):		
Angel Flake	⅓ cup	118
Cookie	⅓ cup	186
Premium shred	⅓ cup	138
(Durkee) shredded	¼ cup	69
COCO WHEATS, cereal	1 T.	44
COD:		
Broiled	3 oz.	145
Frozen (Van de Kamp's)		
Today's Catch	4-oz. serving	80
COD DINNER OR ENTREE, frozen (Armour) *Dinner Classics,* almondine	12-oz. dinner	360
COFFEE:		
Regular:		
*Max-Pax; Maxwell House Electra Perk; Yuban, Yuban Electra Matic	6 fl. oz.	2
*Mellow Roast	6 fl.oz.	8
Decaffeinated:		
*Brim, regular or electric perk	6 fl. oz.	2

Food and Description	Measure or Quantity	Calories
*Brim, freeze-dried; *Decafé;* *Nescafé*	6 fl. oz.	4
*Sanka, regular or electric perk	6 fl. oz.	2
*Instant:		
Maxwell House; Taster's Choice	6 fl. oz.	4
Mellow Roast	6 fl. oz.	8
Sunrise	6 fl. oz.	6
*Mix (General Foods)		
International Coffee:		
Café Amaretto, Café Français	6 fl. oz.	59
Café Vienna, Orange Cappuccino	6 fl. oz.	65
Suisse Mocha	6 fl. oz.	58
COFFEE CAKE (See CAKE, Coffee)		
COFFEE LIQUEUR (DeKuyper)	1½ fl. oz.	140
COFFEE SOUTHERN	1 fl. oz.	79
COGNAC (See **DISTILLED LIQUOR**)		
COLA SOFT DRINK		
(See SOFT DRINK, Cola)		
COLD DUCK WINE		
(Great Western) pink	3 fl. oz.	92
COLESLAW, solids & liq.,		
made with mayonnaise-type		
salad dressing	1 cup	119
*COLESLAW MIX** (Libby's)		
Super Slaw	½ cup	240
COLLARDS:		
Leaves, cooked	⅓ pkg.	31
Canned (Allen's) chopped,		
solids & liq.	½ cup	25
Frozen:		
(Birds Eye) chopped	⅓ pkg.	30
(McKenzie) chopped	⅓ pkg.	25
(Southland) chopped	⅕ of 16-oz. pkg.	25
COMPLETE CEREAL (Elam's)	1 oz.	109
CONCORD WINE:		
(Gold Seal)	3 fl. oz.	125
(Pleasant Valley) red	3 fl. oz.	90
COOKIE, REGULAR:		
Almond Supreme (Pepperidge		
Farm)	1 piece	70
Animal:		
(Dixie Belle)	1 piece	8
(Nabisco) *Barnum's Animals*	1 piece	12
(Sunshine)	1 piece	8
(Tom's)	½ oz.	62
Apricot Raspberry		
(Pepperidge Farm)	1 piece	50
Assortment:		
(Nabisco) *Mayfair:*		
Crown creme sandwich	1 piece	53
Fancy shortbread biscuit	1 piece	22
Filigree creme sandwich	1 piece	60

Food and Description	Measure or Quantity	Calories
Mayfair creme sandwich	1 piece	65
Tea rose creme	1 piece	53
(Pepperidge Farm):		
Butter	1 piece	55
Champagne	1 piece	32
Chocolate lace & Pirouette	1 piece	37
Seville	1 piece	55
Southport	1 piece	75
Blueberry (Pepperidge Farm)	1 piece	57
Blueberry Newtons (Nabisco)	1 piece	73
Bordeaux (Pepperidge Farm)	1 piece	33
Brown edge wafer (Nabisco)	1 piece	28
Brownie:		
(Hostess)	1.25-oz. piece	157
(Nabisco) *Almost Home*	1¼-oz. piece	160
(Pepperidge Farm) chocolate nut	.4-oz. piece	57
Brussels (Pepperidge Farm)	1 piece	53
Brussels Mint (Pepperidge Farm)	1 piece	67
Butter (Sunshine)	1 piece	30
Cappucino (Pepperidge Farm)	1 piece	53
Chessman (Pepperidge Farm)	1 piece	43
Chocolate & chocolate-covered:		
(Keebler) stripes	1 piece	50
(Nabisco):		
Pinwheel, cake	1 piece	130
Snap	1 piece	19
(Sunshine) nuggets	1 piece	23
Chocolate chip:		
(Keebler) Rich 'n Chips	1 piece	80
(Nabisco):		
Almost Home	1 piece	65
Chips Ahoy!		
Regular	1 piece	47
Chewy	1 piece	65
Snaps	1 piece	22
(Pepperidge Farm):		
Regular	1 piece	50
Chocolate	1 piece	53
Mocha	1 piece	40
(Sunshine):		
Chip-A-Roos	1 piece	60
Chippy Chews	1 piece	50
(Tom's)	1.7-oz. serving	230
Date Nut Granola (Pepperidge Farm)	1 piece	53
Fig bar:		
(Nabisco) *Fig Newtons*	1 piece	50
(Sunshine) Chewies	1 piece	50
(Tom's)	1.8-oz. serving	170
Fruit Stick (Nabisco) *Almost Home*	1 piece	70
Gingerman (Pepperidge Farm)	1 piece	57
Ginger Snap:		
(Nabisco)	1 piece	30

Food and Description	Measure or Quantity	Calories
(Sunshine)	1 piece	20
Golden Fruit Raisin (Sunshine)	1 piece	70
Hazelnut (Pepperidge Farm)	1 piece	57
Ladyfinger	3¼″ × 1⅜″ × 1⅛″	40
Lido (Pepperidge Farm)	1 piece	95
Macaroon, coconut (Nabisco)	1 piece	95
Mallow Puffs (Sunshine)	1 piece	70
Marshmallow:		
(Nabisco):		
Mallomars	1 piece	65
Puffs, cocoa covered	1 piece	120
Sandwich	1 piece	30
Twirls cakes	1 piece	130
(Planters) banana pie	1 oz.	127
Milano (Pepperidge Farm)	1 piece	60
Mint Milano (Pepperidge Farm)	1 piece	76
Molasses (Nabisco) *Pantry*	1 piece	65
Molasses Crisp (Pepperidge Farm)	1 piece	33
Nilla wafer (Nabisco)	1 piece	19
Oatmeal:		
(Keebler) old fashioned	1 piece	80
(Nabisco) *Bakers Bonus*	1 piece	65
(Pepperidge Farm):		
Irish	1 piece	47
Raisin	1 piece	57
(Sunshine) Country	1 piece	60
Orange Milano (Pepperidge Farm)	1 piece	76
Orbits (Sunshine)	1 piece	15
Peanut & peanut butter (Nabisco):		
Almost Home	1 piece	70
Nutter Butter, sandwich	1 piece	70
Pecan Sandies (Keebler)	1 piece	80
Raisin:		
(Nabisco) *Almost Home:*		
Fudge chocolate chip	1 piece	65
Iced applesauce	1 piece	70
(Pepperidge Farm) bran	1 piece	53
Raisin Bran (Pepperidge Farm) *Kitchen Hearth*	1 piece	53
Sandwich:		
(Keebler):		
Fudge creme	1 piece	60
Pitter Patter	1 piece	90
(Nabisco):		
Regular:		
Baronet	1 piece	47
Gaity	1 piece	50
Giggles	1 piece	70
I Screams	1 piece	75
Oreo, regular	1 piece	47
Almost Home	1 piece	140

Food and Description	Measure or Quantity	Calories
(Sunshine):		
Regular, *Hydrox*	1 piece	50
Chips 'n Middles	1 piece	70
Tru Blu	1 piece	80
Shortbread or shortcake:		
(Nabisco):		
Lorna Doone	1 piece	35
Pecan	1 piece	75
(Pepperidge Farm)	1 piece	75
Social Tea, biscuit (Nabisco)	1 piece	22
Sprinkles (Sunshine)	1 piece	70
Sugar cookie (Nabisco) rings, *Bakers Bonus*	1 piece	65
Sugar wafer:		
(Dutch Twin) any flavor	1 piece	36
(Nabisco) *Biscos*	1 piece	19
(Sunshine)	1 piece	45
Tahiti (Pepperidge Farm)	1 piece	85
Toy (Sunshine)	1 piece	12
Waffle creme (Dutch Twin)	1 piece	45
COOKIE, DIETETIC (Estee):		
Chocolate chip, coconut or oatmeal raisin	1 piece	30
Wafer, chocolate covered	1 piece	120
COOKIE CRISP, cereal, any flavor	1 cup	110
*COOKIE DOUGH:		
Refrigerated (Pillsbury):		
Chocolate chip or sugar	1 cookie	57
Double chocolate or peanut butter	1 cookie	57
Frozen (Rich's):		
Chocolate chip	1 cookie	138
Oatmeal	1 cookie	125
*COOKIE MIX:		
Regular:		
Brownie:		
(Betty Crocker):		
Fudge, regular size	1/16 pan	150
Walnut, family size	1/24 pan	130
(Pillsbury) fudge, regular size	2" sq. (1/16 pkg.)	150
Chocolate chip:		
(Betty Crocker) *Big Batch*	1 cookie	60
(Duncan Hines)	1/36 pkg.	72
(Nestlé)	1 cookie	60
(Quaker)	1 cookie	75
Fudge chip (Quaker)	1 cookie	75
Macaroon, coconut (Betty Crocker)	1/24 pkg.	80
Oatmeal:		
(Betty Crocker) *Big Batch*	1 cookie	65
(Quaker)	1 cookie	66

46

Food and Description	Measure or Quantity	Calories
Peanut butter (Duncan Hines)	1/36 pkg.	68
Sugar:		
(Betty Crocker) *Big Batch*	1 cookie	60
(Duncan Hines) golden	1 cookie	59
Dietetic (Estee) brownie	2" × 2" sq. cookie	45
COOKING SPRAY, *Mazola No Stick*	2-second spray	8
CORN:		
Fresh, on the cob, boiled	5" × 1¾" ear	70
Canned, regular pack, solids & liq.:		
(Allen's) whole kernel	½ cup	80
(Comstock) whole kernel	½ cup	90
(Del Monte):		
Cream style, golden	½ cup	95
Whole kernel	½ cup	100
(Green Giant):		
Cream style	4¼ oz.	96
Whole kernel, golden	4¼ oz.	79
Whole kernel, *Mexicorn*	3½ oz.	90
(Larsen) *Freshlike,* whole kernel, vacuum pack	½ cup	100
(Libby's) cream style	½ cup	100
(Stokely-Van Camp):		
Cream style	½ cup	105
Whole kernel, solids & liq.	½ cup	74
Canned, dietetic pack, solids & liq.:		
(Del Monte) No Salt Added	½ cup	70
(Diet Delight)	½ cup	60
(Larsen) *Fresh-Lite*	½ cup	80
(S&W) *Nutradiet,* whole kernel, green label	½ cup	80
Frozen:		
(Birds Eye):		
On the cob:		
Farmside	4.4-oz. ear	140
Little Ears	2.3-oz. ear	73
With butter sauce	⅓ pkg.	98
(Frosty Acres):		
On the cob	1 whole ear	120
Kernels	3.3 oz.	80
(Green Giant):		
On the cob:		
Nibbler	2.7-oz. ear	80
Niblet Ear	4.9-oz. ear	140
Whole kernel, *Harvest Fresh*	½ cup	101
Whole kernel, *Niblets,* golden, polybag	⅓ pkg.	80
(Seabrook Farms):		
On the cob	5" ear	140
Whole kernel	⅓ pkg.	97
CORNBREAD:		
Home recipe:		
Corn pone	4 oz.	231

Food and Description	Measure or Quantity	Calories
Spoon bread	4 oz.	221
*Mix:		
(Aunt Jemima)	⅙ pkg.	220
(Dromedary)	2" × 2" piece	130
(Pillsbury) *Ballard*	⅛ of recipe	140
*CORN DOGS, frozen		
(Hormel)	1 piece	220
CORNED BEEF:		
Cooked, boneless, medium fat	4-oz. serving	422
Canned, regular pack:		
Dinty Moore (Hormel)	2-oz. serving	130
(Libby's)	⅓ of 7-oz. can	160
Canned, dietetic (Featherweight)		
loaf	2½-oz. serving	90
Packaged (Carl Buddig) sliced	1-oz. slice	40
CORNED BEEF HASH, canned:		
(Libby's)	⅓ of 24-oz. can	420
Mary Kitchen (Hormel)	7½-oz. serving	360
CORNED BEEF HASH DINNER,		
frozen (Banquet)	10-oz. dinner	372
CORNED BEEF SPREAD		
(Underwood)	½ of 4½-oz. can	120
CORN FLAKE CRUMBS		
(Kellogg's)	¼ cup	110
CORN FLAKES, cereal:		
(General Mills) *Country*	1 cup	110
(Kellogg's) regular	1 cup	110
(Ralston Purina) regular	1 cup	110
CORN MEAL:		
Bolted (Aunt Jemima/Quaker)	3 T.	102
Degermed	¼ cup	125
Mix, bolted (Aunt Jemima) white	1 cup	392
CORN POPS, cereal		
(Kellogg's)	1 cup	110
CORN PUREE (Larsen)	½ cup	100
CORNSTARCH (Argo; Kingsford's; Duryea)	1 tsp.	10
CORN SYRUP (See SYRUP, Corn)		
COUGH DROP:		
(Beech-Nut)	1 drop	10
(Pine Bros.)	1 drop	10
COUNT CHOCULA, cereal		
(General Mills)	1 oz. (1 cup)	110
CRAB:		
Fresh, steamed:		
Whole	½ lb.	101
Meat only	4 oz.	105
Canned, drained	4 oz.	115
Frozen (Wakefield's)	4 oz.	96
CRAB APPLE, flesh only	¼ lb.	71
CRAB APPLE JELLY (Smucker's)	1 T.	53

Food and Description	Measure or Quantity	Calories
CRAB AU GRATIN, frozen (Gorton's) *Light Recipe*	1 package	280
CRAB, DEVILED, frozen (Mrs. Paul's) breaded & fried, regular	½ of 6-oz. pkg.	170
CRAB IMPERIAL, home recipe	1 cup	323
CRACKERS, PUFFS & CHIPS:		
Arrowroot biscuit (Nabisco)	1 piece	22
Bacon-flavored thins (Nabisco)	1 piece	10
Bacon Nips	1 oz.	147
Bran wafer (Featherweight)	1 piece	13
Bravos (Wise)	1 oz.	150
Bugles (Tom's)	1 oz.	150
Cafe (Sunshine)	1 piece	20
Cheese flavored:		
American Heritage (Sunshine):		
Cheddar	1 piece	16
Parmesan	1 piece	18
Better Blue Thins (Nabisco)	1 piece	7
Cheddar sticks (Flavor Tree)	1 oz.	160
Cheese bites (Tom's)	1½ oz.	200
Cheese Doodles (Wise):		
Crunchy	1 oz.	160
Puffed	1 oz.	150
Chee-Tos, crunchy or puffy	1 oz.	160
Cheez Balls (Planters)	1 oz.	160
Cheez Curls (Planters)	1 oz.	160
Cheeze-It (Sunshine)	1 piece	6
Corn Cheese (Tom's) crunchy	1⅝ oz.	280
(Dixie Belle)	1 piece	6
Nacho cheese cracker (Keebler)	1 piece	11
Nips (Nabisco)	1 piece	5
Tid-Bit (Nabisco)	1 piece	4
Chicken in a Biskit (Nabisco)	1 piece	10
Chipsters (Nabisco)	1 piece	2
Club cracker (Keebler)	1 piece	15
Corn chips:		
(Bachman) regular or BBQ	1 oz.	150
Dipsy Doodle (Wise)	1 oz.	160
(Featherweight) low sodium	1 oz.	170
(Flavor Tree)	1 oz.	150
Fritos:		
Regular	1 oz.	160
Barbecue flavor	1 oz.	150
Korkers (Nabisco)	1 piece	8
(Laura Scudder's)	1 oz.	160
(Tom's) regular	1 oz.	155
Creme Wafer Stick (Nabisco)	1 piece	47
Corn Stick (Flavor Tree)	1 oz.	160
Crown Pilot (Nabisco)	1 piece	60
Diggers (Nabisco)	1 piece	4

Food and Description	Measure or Quantity	Calories
English Water Biscuit		
(Pepperidge Farm)	1 piece	17
Escort (Nabisco)	1 piece	27
French onion cracker (Nabisco)	1 piece	12
Goldfish (Pepperidge Farm)		
Tiny	1 piece	3
Graham:		
Cinnamon Crisp (Keebler)	1 piece	17
(Dixie Belle) sugar-honey coated	1 piece	15
Flavor Kist (Schulze and Burch)		
sugar-honey coated	1 piece	57
Honey Maid (Nabisco)	1 piece	30
(Rokeach)	8 pieces	120
(Sunshine) cinnamon	1 piece	17
Graham, chocolate or cocoa-		
covered:		
(Keebler)	1 piece	40
(Nabisco)	1 piece	57
Great Crisps! (Nabisco):		
French onion	1 piece	10
Nacho	1 piece	9
Real bacon or sesame	1 piece	8
Hi Ho (Sunshine)	1 piece	20
Meal Mates (Nabisco)	1 piece	23
Melba Toast (See MELBA TOAST)		
Milk Lunch Biscuit (Keebler)	1 piece	27
Mucho Macho Nacho, Flavor Kist		
(Schulze and Burch)	1 oz.	121
Nachips (Old El Paso)	1 piece	17
Nacho Rings (Tom's)	1 oz.	160
Onion rings (Wise)	1 oz.	130
Oyster:		
(Dixie Belle)	1 piece	4
(Keebler) *Zesta*	1 piece	2
(Nabisco) *Dandy* or *Oysterettes*	1 piece	3
(Sunshine)	1 piece	4
Party (Estee)	½ oz.	70
Party mix (Flavor Tree)	1 oz.	160
Pizza Crunchies (Planters)	1 oz.	160
Ritz (Nabisco)	1 piece	17
Roman Meal Wafer, boxed	1 piece	11
Royal Lunch (Nabisco)	1 piece	60
Rusk, *Holland* (Nabisco)	1 piece	60
Rye toast (Keebler)	1 piece	16
RyKrisp:		
Natural	1 triple cracker	25
Seasoned or sesame	1 triple cracker	30
Saltine:		
(Dixie Belle) regular or unsalted	1 piece	12
Krispy (Sunshine)	1 piece	12
Premium (Nabisco)	1 piece	12

Food and Description	Measure or Quantity	Calories
(Rokeach)	1 piece	12
Zesta (Keebler)	1 piece	12
Sea Toast (Keebler)	1 piece	60
Sesame:		
American Heritage (Sunshine)	1 piece	17
Butter flavored (Nabisco)	1 piece	17
Chip (Flavor Tree)	1 oz.	150
Crunch (Flavor Tree)	1 oz.	150
(Estee)	½ oz.	70
Stick (Flavor Tree):		
Regular	1 oz.	150
With bran or low sodium	1 oz.	160
Toast (Keebler)	1 piece	16
Skittle Chips (Nabisco)	1 piece	14
Snackers (Ralston)	1 piece	17
Snackin Crisp (Durkee) *D&C*	1 oz.	155
Snacks Sticks (Pepperidge Farm):		
Cheese	1 piece	17
Lightly salted, pumpernickel, rye & sesame	1 piece	16
Sociables (Nabisco)	1 piece	12
Sour cream-onion stick (Flavor Tree)	1 oz.	150
Spirals (Wise)	1 oz.	160
Table Water Cracker (Carr's) small	1 piece	15
Taco chip (Laura Scudder's)	1 oz.	150
Tortilla chips:		
(Bachman) nacho, taco flavor or toasted	1 oz.	140
Doritos, nacho or taco	1 oz.	140
(Laura Scudder's)	1 oz.	140
(Nabisco) regular and nacho	1 piece	11
(Planters)	1 oz.	150
(Tom's)	1½ oz.	210
Town House Cracker (Keebler)	1 piece	16
Triscuit (Nabisco)	1 piece	20
Tuc (Keebler)	1 piece	23
Twigs (Nabisco)	1 piece	14
Uneeda Biscuit (Nabisco) unsalted	1 piece	20
Unsalted (Featherweight)	2 sections (½ cracker)	30
Waverly (Nabisco)	1 piece	17
Wheat (Pepperidge Farm) cracked or hearty	1 piece	25
Wheatmeal Biscuit (Carr's) small	1 piece	42
Wheat Nuts (Flavor Tree)	1 oz.	200
Wheat Snack (Dixie Belle)	1 piece	9
Wheat Snaz (Estee)	1 oz.	110
Wheatsworth (Nabisco)	1 piece	14
Wheat Thins (Nabisco) cheese	1 piece	9
Wheat Toast (Keebler)	1 piece	15

Food and Description	Measure or Quantity	Calories
Wheat wafer (Featherweight) unsalted	1 piece	13
CRACKER CRUMBS, graham:		
(Nabisco)	2 T.	80
(Sunshine)	½ cup	275
CRACKER MEAL (Nabisco)	2 T.	50
CRANAPPLE JUICE (Ocean Spray) canned:		
Regular	6 fl. oz.	129
Dietetic	6 fl. oz.	32
CRANBERRY, fresh (Ocean Spray)	½ cup	26
CRANBERRY-APPLE JUICE COCKTAIL, frozen (Welch's)	6 fl. oz.	120
CRANBERRY JUICE COCKTAIL:		
Canned (Ocean Spray):		
Regular	6 fl. oz.	106
Dietetic	6 fl. oz.	36
*Frozen (Welch's)	6 fl. oz.	100
CRANBERRY-ORANGE RELISH (Ocean Spray)	2 oz.	104
CRANBERRY-RASPBERRY SAUCE (Ocean Spray) jellied	2 oz.	89
CRANBERRY SAUCE:		
Home recipe, sweetened, unstrained	4 oz.	202
Canned (Ocean Spray):		
Jellied	2 oz.	88
Whole berry	2 oz.	89
CRANGRAPE (Ocean Spray)	6 fl. oz.	108
CRANRASPBERRY (Ocean Spray)	6 fl. oz.	110
CRANTASTIC JUICE DRINK, canned (Ocean Spray)	6 fl. oz.	110
CRAZY COW, cereal (General Mills)	1 cup	110
CREAM:		
Half & half (Dairylea)	1 fl. oz.	40
Heavy whipping (Dairylea)	1 fl. oz.	60
Light, table or coffee (Sealtest) 16% fat	1 T.	26
Light, whipping, 30% fat (Sealtest)	1 T.	45
Sour (Dairylea)	1 fl. oz.	60
Sour, imitation (Pet)	1 T.	25
Substitute (See CREAM SUBSTITUTE)		
CREAM PUFFS:		
Home recipe, custard filling	3½" × 2" piece	303
Frozen (Rich's) chocolate	1⅓-oz. piece	146
CREAM OF RICE, cereal	1 oz.	100
CREAMSICLE (Popsicle Industries)	2½-fl.-oz. piece	80
CREAM SUBSTITUTE:		
Coffee Mate (Carnation)	1 tsp.	11
Cremora (Borden)	1 tsp.	12
Dairy Light (Alba)	2.8-oz. envelope	10
N-Rich	3-gram packet	16

52

Food and Description	Measure or Quantity	Calories
(Pet)	1 tsp.	10
CREAM OF WHEAT, cereal:		
Regular	1 oz.	100
*Instant	1 oz.	100
*Mix'n Eat:		
Regular	1 packet	100
Apple & cinnamon	1 packet	130
Maple & brown sugar	1 packet	130
Quick	1 T.	40
CREME DE BANANA LIQUEUR		
(Mr. Boston)	1 fl. oz.	93
CREME DE CACAO:		
(Hiram Walker)	1 fl. oz.	104
(Mr. Boston):		
Brown	1 fl. oz.	102
White	1 fl. oz.	93
CREME DE CASSIS (Mr. Boston)	1 fl. oz.	85
CREME DE MENTHE:		
(Bols)	1 fl. oz.	122
(Mr. Boston):		
Green	1 fl. oz.	109
White	1 fl. oz.	97
CREME DE NOYAUX (Mr. Boston)	1 fl. oz.	99
CREPE, frozen:		
(Mrs. Paul's):		
Crab	5½-oz. pkg.	248
Shrimp	5½-oz. pkg.	252
(Stouffer's):		
Chicken with mushroom sauce	8¼-oz. pkg.	390
Spinach with cheddar cheese sauce	9½-oz. pkg.	415
CRISP RICE CEREAL:		
(Featherweight) low sodium	1 cup	110
(Ralston Purina)	1 cup	110
CRISPY WHEATS'N RAISINS, cereal (General Mills)	¾ cup	110
CROUTON:		
(Arnold):		
Bavarian or English style	½ oz.	65
French, Italian or Mexican style	½ oz.	66
(Kellogg's) *Croutettes*	⅔ cup	70
(Pepperidge Farm)	.5 oz.	70
C-3PO'S, cereal (Kellogg's)	¾ cup	110
CUCUMBER:		
Eaten with skin	8-oz. cucumber	32
Pared	7½" × 2"	29
Pared,	3 slices (.9 oz.)	4
CUMIN SEED (French's)	1 tsp.	7
CUPCAKE:		
Regular (Hostess):		
Chocolate	1 cupcake	170

Food and Description	Measure or Quantity	Calories
Orange	1 cupcake	150
Frozen (Sara Lee) yellow	1 cupcake	190
*CUPCAKE MIX (Flako)	1 cupcake	150
CUP O'NOODLES (Nissin Foods):		
Beef	2½-oz. serving	343
Beef onion	2½-oz. serving	323
Chicken	2½-oz. serving	343
Chicken, twin pack	1.2-oz. serving	155
Shrimp	2½-oz. serving	336
CURAÇAO:		
(Bols)	1 fl. oz.	105
(Hiram Walker)	1 fl. oz.	96
CURRANT, DRIED (Del Monte)		
Zante	½ cup	204
CUSTARD:		
Canned (Thank You Brand) egg	½ cup	135
Chilled, *Swiss Miss,* chocolate or egg flavor	4-oz. container	150
*Mix, dietetic (Featherweight)	½ cup	80
C. W. POST, cereal:		
Plain	¼ cup	131
With raisins	¼ cup	128

D

Food and Description	Measure or Quantity	Calories
DAIQUIRI COCKTAIL		
(Mr. Boston):		
Regular	3 fl. oz.	99
Strawberry	3 fl. oz.	111
*DAIQUIRI COCKTAIL MIX		
(Bar-Tender's)	3½ fl. oz.	177
DAIRY CRISP, cereal (Pet)	¼ cup	120
DAIRY QUEEN/BRAZIER:		
Banana split	13.5-oz. serving	540
Brownie Delight, hot fudge	9.4-oz. serving	600
Buster Bar	5¼-oz. piece	460
Chicken sandwich	7.8-oz. sandwich	670
Cone:		
Plain, any flavor, regular	5-oz. cone	240
Dipped, chocolate, regular	5½-oz. cone	340
Dilly Bar	3-oz. piece	210
Double Delight	9-oz. serving	490
DQ Sandwich	2.1-oz. sandwich	140
Fish sandwich:		
Plain	6-oz. sandwich	400
With cheese	6¼-oz. sandwich	440
Float	14-oz. serving	410

Food and Description	Measure or Quantity	Calories
Freeze, vanilla	12-oz. serving	500
French fries:		
Regular	2½-oz. serving	200
Large	4-oz. serving	320
Frozen dessert	4-oz. serving	180
Hamburger:		
Plain:		
Single	5.2-oz. burger	360
Double	7.4-oz. burger	530
Triple	9.6-oz. burger	710
With cheese:		
Single	5.7-oz. burger	410
Double	8.4-oz. burger	650
Triple	10.63-oz. burger	820
Hot dog:		
Regular:		
Plain	3.5-oz. serving	280
With cheese	4-oz. serving	330
With chili	4½-oz. serving	320
Super:		
Plain	6.2-oz. serving	520
With cheese	6.9-oz. serving	580
With chili	7.7-oz. serving	570
Malt, chocolate:		
Large	20¾-oz. serving	1060
Regular	14¾-oz. serving	760
Small	10¼-oz. serving	520
Mr. Misty:		
Plain:		
Large	15½-oz. serving	340
Regular	11.64-oz. serving	250
Small	8¼-oz. serving	190
Kiss	3.14-oz. serving	70
Float	14.5-oz. serving	390
Freeze	14.5-oz. serving	500
Onion rings	3-oz. serving	280
Parfait	10-oz. serving	430
Peanut Butter Parfait	10¾-oz. serving	750
Shake, chocolate:		
Large	20¾-oz. serving	990
Regular	14¾-oz. serving	710
Small	10¼-oz. serving	490
Strawberry shortcake	11-oz. serving	540
Sundae, chocolate:		
Large	8¾-oz. serving	440
Regular	6¼-oz. serving	310
Small	3¾-oz. serving	190
Tomato	½ oz.	4
DATE (Dromedary):		
Chopped	¼ cup	130
Pitted	5 dates	100

Food and Description	Measure or Quantity	Calories
DE CHAUNAC WINE		
(Great Western) 12% alcohol	3 fl. oz.	71
DELI'S, frozen (Pepperidge Farm):		
Mexican style	4-oz. piece	280
Reuben in rye pastry	4-oz. piece	360
Turkey, ham & cheese	4-oz. piece	270
DESSERT CUPS (Hostess)	¾-oz. piece	62
DILL SEED (French's)	1 tsp.	9
DING DONG (Hostess)	1 cake	172
DINNER, frozen (See individual listings such as BEEF, CHICKEN, TURKEY, etc.)		
DIP:		
Acapulco (Ortega) with cheddar cheese	1 oz.	64
Avocado (Nalley's)	1 oz.	114
Bacon & horseradish (Kraft)	1 T.	30
Bacon & onion (Nalley's)	1 oz.	113
Barbecue (Nalley's)	1 oz.	114
Blue cheese:		
(Dean) tang	1 oz.	61
(Nalley's)	1 oz.	110
Clam (Nalley's)	1 oz.	101
Cucumber & onion (Breakstone)	1 oz.	50
Guacamole (Nalley's)	1 oz.	114
Jalapeño:		
Fritos	1 oz.	34
(Hain) natural	1 oz.	40
Onion (Thank You Brand)	1 T.	45
Onion bean (Hain) natural	1 oz.	41
Taco (Thank You Brand)	1 T.	44
DIP 'UM SAUCE, canned (French's):		
BBQ	1 T.	22
Hot mustard	1 T.	35
Sweet 'n sour	1 T.	40
DISTILLED LIQUOR, any brand:		
80 proof	1 fl. oz.	65
86 proof	1 fl. oz.	70
90 proof	1 fl. oz.	74
94 proof	1 fl. oz.	77
100 proof	1 fl. oz.	83
DONUTZ, cereal (General Mills)	1 cup	120
DOUGHNUT (See also *WINCHELL'S*):		
Regular (Hostess):		
Chocolate coated	1-oz. piece	130
Cinnamon	1-oz. piece	110
Donettes, powdered	1 piece	40
Old fashioned, plain	1.5-oz. piece	180
Powdered	1-oz. piece	110

Food and Description	Measure or Quantity	Calories
Frozen (Morton):		
Regular:		
Boston creme	2-oz. piece	180
Chocolate iced	1.5-oz. piece	150
Jelly	1.8-oz. piece	180
Donut Holes	⅓ of 7¾-oz. pkg.	160
Morning Light, jelly	2.6-oz. piece	250
DRAMBUIE (Hiram Walker)	1 fl. oz.	110
DRUMSTICK, frozen:		
Ice cream, in a cone:		
Topped with peanuts	1 piece	181
Topped with peanuts & cone bisque	1 piece	168
Ice milk, in a cone:		
Topped with peanuts	1 piece	163
Topped with peanuts & cone bisque	1 piece	150
DULCITO, frozen (Hormel) apple	4 oz.	290
DUMPLINGS, canned, dietetic (Dia-Mel)	8-oz. serving	160

E

ECLAIR:		
Home recipe, with custard filling and chocolate icing	4-oz. piece	271
Frozen (Rich's) chocolate	1 piece	234
EEL, smoked, meat only	4 oz.	374
EGG, CHICKEN:		
Raw:		
White only	1 large egg	17
Yolk only	1 large egg	59
Boiled	1 large egg	81
Fried in butter	1 large egg	99
Omelet, mixed with milk & cooked in fat	1 large egg	107
Poached	1 large egg	78
Scrambled, mixed with milk & cooked in fat	1 large egg	111
EGG DINNER OR ENTREE, frozen (Swanson):		
Omelet, Spanish style	7¾-oz. meal	250
Scrambled, with sausage & potatoes	6¼-oz. meal	410
***EGG FOO YUNG,** dinner (Chun King) stir fry	5 oz.	138

Food and Description	Measure or Quantity	Calories
EGG MIX (Durkee):		
Omelet:		
*With bacon	½ pkg.	310
*Puffy	½ pkg.	302
Scrambled:		
Plain	.8-oz. pkg.	124
With bacon	1.3-oz. pkg.	181
EGG NOG, dairy (Meadow Gold)		
6% fat	½ cup	164
EGG NOG COCKTAIL		
(Mr. Boston) 15% alcohol	3 fl. oz.	177
EGGPLANT:		
Boiled, drained	4 oz.	22
Frozen:		
(Celentano) rollettes	11-oz. pkg.	420
(Mrs. Paul's):		
Parmesan	5½-oz. serving	270
Sticks, breaded & fried	3½-oz. serving	240
(Weight Watchers) Parmesan	13-oz. pkg.	285
EGG ROLL, frozen:		
(Chun King):		
Chicken	.65-oz. piece	37
Meat & shrimp	2.6-oz. piece	151
Shrimp	.8-oz. piece	41
(La Choy):		
Chicken	.4-oz. piece	30
Lobster	.4-oz. piece	27
Meat & shrimp	.25-oz. piece	17
EGG ROLL DINNER, frozen		
(Van de Kamp's) Cantonese	10½-oz. serving	560
EGG SUBSTITUTE:		
Egg Magic (Featherweight)	½ envelope	60
Scramblers (Morningstar Farms)	1 egg substitute	35
Second Nature (Avoset)	3 T.	42
ENCHILADA OR ENCHILADA DINNER, frozen:		
Beef:		
(Banquet):		
Dinner	12-oz. meal	497
Entree	2-lb. pkg	1056
(Green Giant) Sonora style	12-oz. entree	700
(Hormel)	1 enchilada	140
(Morton)	11-oz. dinner	280
(Van de Kamp's):		
Dinner, regular	12-oz. dinner	390
Entree, shredded	5½-oz. serving	180
Cheese:		
(Banquet)	12-oz. dinner	543
(Van de Kamp's)	12-oz. dinner	450
Chicken (Van de Kamp's)	7½-oz. pkg.	250

58

Food and Description	Measure or Quantity	Calories
ENCHILADA SAUCE:		
Canned:		
(Del Monte) hot or mild	½ cup	45
Old El Paso, hot	¼ cup	27
*Mix (Durkee)	½ cup	29
ENDIVE, CURLY OR ESCAROLE, cut	½ cup	7
ESPRESSO COFFEE LIQUEUR	1 fl. oz.	104

F

Food and Description	Measure or Quantity	Calories
FARINA:		
(Hi-O) dry, regular	1 T.	40
Malt-O-Meal, dry:		
Regular	1 oz.	96
Quick cooking	1 oz.	100
*(Pillsbury) made with milk and salt	⅔ cup	200
FAT, COOKING:		
Crisco:		
Regular	1 T.	110
Butter flavor	1 T.	126
(Rokeach) neutral nyafat	1 T.	99
Spry	1 T.	94
FENNEL SEED (French's)	1 tsp.	8
FETTUCINI ALFREDO, frozen (Stouffer's)	½ of 10-oz. pkg.	270
FIG:		
Small	1½" fig	30
Canned, regular pack (Del Monte) whole, solids & liq.	½ cup	100
Dried (Sun-Maid), Calimyrna	½ cup	250
FIG JUICE (Sunsweet)	6 fl. oz.	120
FIGURINES (Pillsbury) all flavors	1 bar	138
FILBERT:		
Shelled	1 oz.	180
(Fisher) oil dipped, salted	½ cup	360
FISH CAKE, frozen (Mrs. Paul's):		
Breaded & fried	2-oz. piece	110
Thins, breaded & fried	½ of 10-oz. pkg.	300
FISH & CHIPS, frozen:		
(Gorton's)	1 pkg.	1350
(Swanson):		
Regular	5½-oz. entree	320
Hungry Man	14¾-oz. dinner	770
(Van de Kamp's) batter dipped, french fried	7-oz. pkg.	440
FISH DINNER, frozen:		
(Banquet)	8¾-oz. dinner	553

Food and Description	Measure or Quantity	Calories
(Morton)	10-oz. dinner	320
(Mrs. Paul's) Parmesan	½ of 10-oz. pkg.	220
(Stouffer's) *Lean Cuisine*, Florentine	9-oz. pkg.	230
(Weight Watchers):		
Au gratin	9½-oz. meal	200
Oven fried	6¾-oz. meal	220
FISH FILLET, frozen:		
(Gorton's):		
Regular, crunchy	1 piece	175
Light Recipe, tempura batter	1 piece	190
(Mrs. Paul's):		
Batter fried, crunchy	2¼-oz. piece	155
Breaded & fried, light & natural	1 piece	290
(Van de Kamp's):		
Batter dipped, french fried	3-oz. piece	180
Country seasoned	2-oz. piece	200
FISH KABOBS, frozen:		
(Mrs. Paul's) light batter	⅓ pkg.	200
(Van de Kamp's) batter dipped, french fried	4-oz. piece	240
FISH SEASONING (Featherweight)	¼ tsp.	<1
FISH STICKS, frozen:		
(Gorton's) potato crisp	1 piece	60
(Mrs. Paul's):		
Batter fried	1 piece	69
Breaded & fried	1 piece	43
(Van de Kamp's) batter dipped, french fried	1-oz. piece	55
FIT'N FROSTY (Alba '77):		
Chocolate or marshmallow flavor	1 envelope	70
Strawberry	1 envelope	74
Vanilla	1 envelope	69
*****FIVE ALIVE** (Snow Crop)	6 fl. oz.	85
FLOUNDER:		
Baked	4 oz.	229
Frozen:		
(Gorton's) *Fishmarket Fresh*	4 oz.	90
(Mrs. Paul's) fillets, breaded & fried, crispy, crunchy	2-oz. piece	140
FLOUNDER DINNER OR ENTREE, frozen (Le Menu)	10½-oz. dinner	340
FLOUR:		
(Aunt Jemima) self-rising	¼ cup	109
Ballard, self-rising	¼ cup	100
Bisquick (Betty Crocker)	¼ cup	120
(Elam's):		
Brown rice, whole grain	¼ cup	146
Buckwheat, pure	¼ cup	92
Pastry	1 oz.	102

Food and Description	Measure or Quantity	Calories
Rye, whole grain	¼ cup	89
Soy	1 oz.	98
Gold Medal (Betty Crocker)		
all-purpose or high protein	¼ cup	100
La Pina	¼ cup	100
Pillsbury's Best:		
All-purpose or rye, medium	¼ cup	100
Sauce & gravy	2 T.	50
Self-rising	¼ cup	95
Presto, self-rising	¼ cup	98
Wondra	¼ cup	100
FOOD STICKS (Pillsbury) chocolate	1 piece	45
FRANKEN*BERRY, cereal		
(General Mills)	1 cup	110
FRANKFURTER:		
(Eckrich):		
Beef, or meat	1.6-oz. frankfurter	150
Beef or meat, jumbo	2-oz. frankfurter	190
Meat	1.2-oz. frankfurter	120
(Hormel):		
Beef	1.6-oz. frankfurter	139
Range Brand, Wrangler, smoked	1 frankfurter	160
(Hygrade) beef, *Ball Park*	2-oz. frankfurter	169
(Louis Rich) turkey	1.5-oz. frankfurter	95
(Oscar Mayer):		
Bacon & cheddar	1.6-oz. frankfurter	143
Beef	1.6-oz. frankfurter	145
Cheese:		
Regular	1.6-oz. frankfurter	145
Nacho	1.6-oz. frankfurter	138
Little Wiener	2″ frankfurter	28
Wiener	1.6-oz. frankfurter	145
FRANKS-N-BLANKETS, frozen		
(Durkee)	1 piece	45
FRENCH TOAST, frozen:		
(Aunt Jemima):		
Regular	1 slice	85
Cinnamon swirl	1 slice	97
(Swanson) with sausage, plain	6½-oz. meal	450
FRITTERS, frozen (Mrs. Paul's):		
Apple	2-oz. piece	125
Clam	1.9-oz. piece	131
Corn	2-oz. piece	73
Shrimp	½ of 7¾-oz. pkg.	242
FROOT LOOPS, cereal (Kellogg's)	1 cup	110
FROSTED RICE, cereal (Kellogg's)	1 cup	110
FROSTS (Libby's):		
Dry:		
Banana	.5 oz.	50
Orange, strawberry or pineapple	.5 oz.	60
Liquid:		
Banana	7 fl. oz.	120

Food and Description	Measure or Quantity	Calories
Orange or strawberry	8 fl. oz.	120
FROZEN DESSERT, dietetic (See also *TOFUTTI*):		
(Baskin-Robbins)		
Special Diet	1 scoop (2½ fl. oz.)	90
Eskimo, bar, chocolate covered	2½-fl.-oz. bar	110
(SugarLo) all flavors	¼ pt.	135
FRUIT BITS, dried (Sun-Maid)	1 oz.	90
FRUIT COCKTAIL:		
Canned, regular pack, solids & liq.:		
(Del Monte) regular or chunky	½ cup	94
(Libby's)	½ cup	101
(Stokely-Van Camp)	½ cup	95
Canned, dietetic or low calorie, solids & liq.:		
(Del Monte) Lite	½ cup	58
(Diet Delight):		
Syrup pack	½ cup	50
Water pack	½ cup	40
(Featherweight):		
Juice pack	½ cup	50
Water pack	½ cup	40
(Libby's) water pack	½ cup	50
(S&W) *Nutradiet:*		
Juice pack	½ cup	50
Water pack	½ cup	40
FRUIT COMPOTE (Rokeach)	½ cup	120
FRUIT COUNTRY (Comstock):		
Apple or blueberry	¼ pkg.	160
Cherry	¼ pkg.	180
FRUIT CUP (Del Monte):		
Mixed fruits	5-oz. container	110
Peaches, diced	5-oz. container	116
FRUIT, MIXED:		
Canned (Del Monte) lite, chunky	½ cup	58
Frozen (Birds Eye) quick thaw	5-oz. serving	150
FRUIT & FIBER CEREAL (Post)	½ cup	103
FRUIT JUICE, canned (Sun-Maid)	6 fl. oz.	100
FRUIT 'N APPLE JUICE (Tree Top)	6 fl. oz.	90
FRUIT 'N GRAPE JUICE (Tree Top):		
Canned	6 fl. oz.	100
*Frozen	6 fl. oz.	110
FRUIT 'N JUICE BAR (Dole)	2½-fl.-oz. bar	70
FRUIT & NUT MIX (Carnation):		
All fruit	.9-oz. pouch	80
Deluxe trail mix or raisins & nuts	.9-oz. pouch	130
Tropical fruit & nuts	.9-oz. pouch	100
FRUIT PUNCH:		
Canned:		
Capri Sun	6¾ fl. oz.	102

Food and Description	Measure or Quantity	Calories
(Hi-C)	6 fl. oz.	93
(Lincoln)	6 fl. oz.	90
Chilled:		
Five Alive (Snow Crop)	6 fl. oz.	87
(Sunkist)	8.45 fl. oz.	140
*Frozen, *Five Alive* (Snow Crop)	6 fl. oz.	87
*Mix (Hi-C)	6 fl. oz.	72
FRUIT ROLL:		
(Betty Crocker)	1 piece	50
(Flavor Tree)	¾-oz. roll	80
(Sunkist)	½-oz. piece	50
FRUIT SALAD:		
Canned, regular pack:		
(Del Monte) fruits for salad	½ cup	93
(Libby's)	½ cup	99
Canned, dietetic or low calorie:		
(Diet Delight)	½ cup	60
(Featherweight):		
Juice pack	½ cup	50
Water pack	½ cup	40
(S&W) *Nutradiet:*		
Juice pack	½ cup	60
Water pack	½ cup	35
FRUIT SQUARES, frozen		
(Pepperidge Farm)	2½-oz. piece	230
FUDGSICLE (Popsicle Industries)	2½-fl.-oz. bar	100

G

GARLIC:		
Flakes (Gilroy)	1 tsp.	5
Powder (French's)	1 tsp.	5
Spread (Lawry's)	1 T.	79
GEFILTE FISH, canned:		
(Mother's):		
Jellied, old world	4-oz. serving	70
Jellied, white fish & pike	4-oz. serving	60
In liquid broth	4-oz. serving	70
(Rokeach):		
Natural Broth	2-oz. serving	46
Old Vienna:		
Regular	2-oz. serving	52
Jelled	2-oz. serving	54
GELATIN, dry, *Carmel Kosher*	7-gram envelope	30
***GELATIN DESSERT MIX:**		
Regular:		
Carmel Kosher, all flavors	½ cup	80

Food and Description	Measure or Quantity	Calories
(Jell-O) all flavors	½ cup	81
Dietetic:		
Carmel Kosher	½ cup	8
(D-Zerta) all flavors	½ cup	6
(Featherweight) artificially		
sweetened or regular	½ cup	10
*(Royal)	½ cup	12
GELATIN, DRINKING (Knox)		
orange	1 envelope	50
GERMAN STYLE DINNER, frozen		
(Swanson)	11¾-oz. dinner	370
GIN, SLOE:		
(Bols)	1 fl. oz.	85
(DeKuyper)	1 fl. oz.	70
(Mr. Boston)	1 fl. oz.	68
GINGER, powder (French's)	1 tsp.	6
GINGERBREAD:		
Home recipe (USDA)	1.9-oz. piece	174
Mix:		
(Betty Crocker)	⅑ of cake	210
(Dromedary)	2″ × 2″ square	100
(Pillsbury)	3″ square	190
GOLDEN GRAHAMS, cereal		
(General Mills)	¾ cup	110
GOOBER GRAPE (Smucker's)	1 T.	90
GOOD HUMOR (See ICE CREAM)		
GOOD N' PUDDIN		
(Popsicle Industries) all flavors	2⅓-fl.-oz. bar	170
GOOSE, roasted, meat & skin	4 oz.	500
GRAHAM CRAKOS, cereal		
(Kellogg's)	1 cup	110
GRANOLA BAR:		
Nature Valley:		
Regular:		
Almond or cinnamon	1 piece	110
Coconut or peanut	1 piece	120
Chewy:		
Apple	1 piece	130
Peanut butter	1 piece	140
New Trail:		
Chocolate chip or peanut butter	1.3-oz. piece	200
Cocoa creme	1.3-oz. piece	90
GRANOLA BAR MIX, chewy,		
Nature Valley, Bake-A-Bar	1 bar	100
GRANOLA CEREAL:		
Nature Valley:		
Cinnamon & raisin, fruit & nut or		
toasted oat	⅓ cup	130
Coconut & honey	⅓ cup	150
Sun Country:		
With almonds	1 oz.	130
With raisins & dates	1 oz.	130

Food and Description	Measure or Quantity	Calories
GRANOLA CLUSTERS,		
Nature Valley:		
Almond	1 piece	140
Caramel & raisin	1 piece	150
GRANOLA & FRUIT BAR,		
Nature Valley	1 bar	150
GRANOLA SNACK:		
Nature Valley	1 pouch	140
Kudos (M&M/Mars):		
Chocolate chip	1¼-oz. piece	180
Peanut butter	1.3-oz. piece	190
Nature Valley	1 piece	140
GRAPE:		
American, ripe (slipskin)	3½″ × 3″ bunch	43
Canned, dietetic (Featherweight)		
light, seedless, water pack	½ cup	60
GRAPE DRINK:		
Canned:		
Capri Sun	6¾ fl. oz.	104
(Hi-C)	6 fl. oz.	89
(Lincoln)	6 fl. oz.	90
(Welchade)	6 fl. oz.	90
Chilled (Sunkist)	8.45 fl. oz.	140
*Frozen (Welchade)	6 fl. oz.	90
*Mix:		
Regular (Hi-C)	6 fl. oz.	68
Dietetic (Sunkist)	8 fl. oz.	6
GRAPEFRUIT:		
Pink & red:		
Seeded type	½ med. grapefruit	46
Seedless type	½ med. grapefruit	49
White:		
Seeded type	½ med. grapefruit	44
Seedless type	½ med. grapefruit	46
Canned, regular pack (Del Monte)		
in syrup	½ cup	74
Canned, dietetic pack, solids & liq.:		
(Del Monte) sections	½ cup	45
(Diet Delight) sections	½ cup	45
(Featherweight) sections,		
juice pack	½ cup	40
(S&W) *Nutradiet*	½ cup	40
GRAPEFRUIT DRINK, canned		
(Lincoln)	6 fl. oz.	104
GRAPEFRUIT JUICE:		
Fresh, pink, red or white	½ cup	46
Canned, sweetened:		
(Del Monte)	6 fl. oz.	89
(Texsun)	6 fl. oz.	77
Canned, unsweetened:		
(Del Monte)	6 fl. oz.	72

Food and Description	Measure or Quantity	Calories
(Ocean Spray)	6 fl. oz.	64
(Texsun)	6 fl. oz.	77
Chilled (Minute Maid)	6 fl. oz.	75
GRAPEFRUIT JUICE COCKTAIL,		
canned (Ocean Spray) pink	6 fl. oz.	84
GRAPEFRUIT-ORANGE JUICE		
COCKTAIL, canned, Musselman's	6 fl. oz.	67
GRAPE JAM (Smucker's)	1 T.	53
GRAPE JELLY:		
Sweetened:		
(Smucker's)	1 T.	53
(Welch's)	1 T.	52
Dietetic:		
(Diet Delight)	1 T.	12
(Estee)	1 T.	6
(Welch's)	1 T.	30
GRAPE JUICE:		
Canned, unsweetened:		
(Seneca Foods)	6 fl. oz.	118
(Tree Top) sparkling	6 fl. oz.	120
(Welch's) regular or red	6 fl. oz.	120
*Frozen:		
(Minute Maid)	6 fl. oz.	99
(Welch's)	6 fl. oz.	100
GRAPE JUICE DRINK, chilled		
(Sunkist)	8.45 fl. oz.	140
GRAPE NUTS, cereal (Post):		
Regular	¼ cup	108
Flakes	⅞ cup	108
Raisin	¼ cup	103
GRAVY, canned:		
Au jus (Franco-American)	2-oz. serving	5
Beef (Franco-American)	2-oz. serving	25
Brown:		
(Estee) dietetic	¼ cup	14
(Franco-American) with onion	2-oz. serving	25
(Howard Johnson's)	½ cup	51
Ready Gravy	¼ cup	44
Chicken (Franco-American):		
Regular	2-oz. serving	50
Giblet	2-oz. serving	26
Chicken & herb	¼ cup	20
Mushroom (Franco-American)	2-oz. serving	25
Pork (Franco-American)	2-oz. serving	40
Turkey:		
(Franco-American)	2-oz. serving	30
(Howard Johnson's) giblet	½ cup	55
GRAVYMASTER	1 tsp.	11
GRAVY MIX:		
Regular:		
Au jus:		
*(Durkee)	½ cup	15

Food and Description	Measure or Quantity	Calories
*(French's) *Gravy Makins*	½ cup	20
Brown:		
*(Durkee) regular	½ cup	29
*(French's) *Gravy Makins*	½ cup	40
*(McCormick)	.85-oz. pkg.	82
*(Pillsbury)	½ cup	30
*(Spatini)	1 oz.	8
Chicken:		
*(Durkee) regular	½ cup	43
*(French's) *Gravy Makins*	½ cup	50
*(Pillsbury)	½ cup	50
Home style:		
*(Durkee)	½ cup	35
*(French's) *Gravy Makins*	½ cup	40
*(Pillsbury)	½ cup	30
Meatloaf (Durkee) *Roasting Bag*	1.5-oz. pkg.	129
Mushroom:		
*(Durkee)	½ cup	30
*(French's) *Gravy Makins*	½ cup	40
Onion:		
*(Durkee)	½ cup	42
*(French's) *Gravy Makins*	½ cup	50
*(McCormick)	.85-oz. pkg.	72
Pork:		
*(Durkee)	½ cup	35
*(French's) *Gravy Makins*	½ cup	40
*Swiss Steak (Durkee)	½ cup	23
Turkey:		
*(Durkee)	½ cup	47
*(French's) *Gravy Makins*	½ cup	50
*Dietetic (Weight Watchers):		
Brown	½ cup	16
Brown, with mushroom	½ cup	24
Brown, with onion	½ cup	26
Chicken	½ cup	20
GRAVY WITH MEAT OR TURKEY,		
Frozen:		
(Banquet):		
Entree for One, & sliced beef	4 oz.	90
Family Entree, & sliced turkey	32-oz. pkg.	640
(Morton) Light, sliced turkey	8 oz.	270
(Swanson) sliced beef	8-oz. entree	200
GREAT BEGINNINGS		
(Hormel):		
With chunky beef	5 oz.	136
With chunky chicken	5 oz.	147
With chunky turkey	5 oz.	138
GREENS, MIXED, canned:		
(Allens)	½ cup	25
(Sunshine) solids & liq.	½ cup	20

Food and Description	Measure or Quantity	Calories
GRENADINE (Garnier) no alcohol	1 fl. oz	103
GUAVA	1 guava	48
GUAVA NECTAR (Libby's)	6 fl. oz.	70

H

Food and Description	Measure or Quantity	Calories
HADDOCK:		
Fried, breaded	4″ × 3″ × ½″ fillet	165
Frozen:		
(Gorton's) *Light Recipe,* fillet entree	1 piece	260
(Mrs. Paul's) breaded & fried crispy, crunchy	2-oz. fillet	140
(Van de Kamp's) batter dipped, french fried	2-oz. piece	120
(Weight Watchers) with stuffing, 2-compartment	7-oz. pkg.	205
Smoked	4-oz. serving	117
HALIBUT:		
Broiled	4″ × 3″ × ½″ steak	214
Frozen (Van de Kamp's) batter dipped, french fried	½ of 8-oz. pkg.	260
HAM:		
Canned:		
(Hormel):		
Black Label (3- or 5-lb. size)	4 oz.	140
Chunk	6¾-oz. serving	310
Patties	1 patty	180
(Oscar Mayer) *Jubilee,* extra lean, cooked	1-oz. serving	31
(Swift) *Premium*	1¾-oz. slice	111
Deviled:		
(Hormel)	1 T.	35
(Libby's)	1 T.	43
(Underwood)	1 T.	49
Packaged:		
(Carl Buddig) smoked	1 oz.	50
(Eckrich):		
Loaf	1 oz.	70
Cooked or imported, Danish	1.2-oz. slice	30
(Hormel):		
Black, or red peppered or frozen	1 slice	25
Chopped	1 slice	55
(Oscar Mayer):		
Chopped	1-oz. slice	64
Cooked, smoked	1-oz. slice	34

Food and Description	Measure or Quantity	Calories
Jubilee, boneless:		
Sliced	8-oz. slice	232
Steak, 95% fat free	2-oz. steak	59
HAM & CHEESE:		
(Eckrich) loaf	1-oz. serving	60
(Hormel) loaf	1-oz. serving	65
HAM DINNER, frozen:		
(Banquet) American Favorites	10-oz. dinner	532
(Morton)	10-oz. dinner	301
HAM SALAD, canned (Carnation)	¼ of 7½-oz. can	110
HAM SALAD SPREAD		
(Oscar Mayer)	1 oz.	62
HAMBURGER (See *McDONALD'S, BURGER KING, DAIRY QUEEN, WHITE CASTLE,* etc.)		
HAMBURGER MIX:		
Hamburger Helper		
(General Mills):		
Beef noodle, tomato or pizza dish	⅓ pkg.	320
Cheeseburger Macaroni	⅓ pkg.	360
Hash	⅓ pkg.	300
Lasagna	⅓ pkg.	330
Potatoes au gratin	⅓ pkg.	320
Stew	⅓ pkg.	290
Make a Better Burger (Lipton)		
mildly seasoned or onion	⅓ pkg.	30
HAMBURGER SEASONING MIX:		
*(Durkee)	1 cup	663
(French's)	1-oz. pkg.	100
HARDEE'S:		
Chef's salad	1 serving	310
Garden salad	1 serving	245
Seafood salad	1 serving	170
Side salad	1 serving	90
Bacon bits	1 packet	15
Crackers	1 packet	35
Croutons	1 packet	30
Blue cheese dressing	1 packet	210
Lo-cal French dressing	1 packet	140
House dressing	1 packet	290
Lo-cal Italian dressing	1 packet	90
Thousand Island dressing	1 packet	250
HAWAIIAN PUNCH:		
Canned regular:		
Cherry or grape	6 fl. oz.	90
Orange	6 fl. oz.	100
Canned, dietetic, punch	6 fl. oz.	30
HEADCHEESE (Oscar Mayer)	1-oz. serving	55
HERRING, canned (Vita):		
Cocktail, drained	8-oz. jar	342
In cream sauce	8-oz. jar	397
Tastee Bits, drained	8-oz. jar	361

Food and Description	Measure or Quantity	Calories
HERRING, SMOKED, kippered	4-oz. serving	239
HICKORY NUT, shelled	1 oz.	191
HO-HO (Hostess)	1-oz. piece	120
HOMINY, canned (Allens) golden, solids & liq.	½ cup	80
HOMINY GRITS:		
Dry:		
(Albers)	1½ oz.	150
(Aunt Jemima)	3 T.	102
(Quaker):		
Regular	3 T.	101
Instant:		
Regular	.8-oz. packet	79
With imitation bacon or ham	1-oz. packet	101
Cooked	1 cup	125
HONEY, strained	1 T.	61
HONEYCOMB, cereal (Post) regular	1⅓ cups	112
HONEYDEW	2" × 7" wedge	31
HONEY SMACKS, cereal (Kellogg's)	¾ cup	110
HORSERADISH:		
Raw, pared	1 oz.	25
Prepared (Gold's)	1 tsp.	3
HOSTESS O'S (Hostess)	2¾-oz. piece	277

I

Food and Description	Measure or Quantity	Calories
ICE CREAM (Listed by type, such as sandwich, or *Whammy,* or by flavor— see also FROZEN DESSERT):		
Almond amaretto (Baskin-Robbins)	4 fl. oz.	280
Bar:		
(Good Humor) vanilla, chocolate coated	3-fl.-oz. piece	170
(Häagen-Dazs):		
Chocolate, dark chocolate coating	1 piece	360
Vanilla, milk chocolate coated	1 bar	330
Bon Bon (Carnation) vanilla	1 piece	33
Brandied black cherry (Häagen-Dazs)	4 fl. oz.	220
Butter Almond (Breyers)	½ cup	170
Butter pecan:		
(Breyer's)	¼ pt.	180
(Good Humor) bulk	4 fl. oz.	150
(Häagen-Dazs)	4 fl. oz.	312
Cappuccino:		
(Baskin-Robbins) chip	4 fl. oz.	310
(Häagen-Dazs)	4 fl. oz.	252
Chocolate:		

Food and Description	Measure or Quantity	Calories
(Baskin-Robbins):		
Regular	4 fl. oz.	264
Mousse Royale	4 fl. oz.	293
(Breyers)	½ cup	160
(Good Humor) bulk	4 fl. oz.	130
(Häagen-Dazs) mint	4 fl. oz.	300
(Howard Johnson's)	½ cup	221
Chocolate chip (Häagen-Dazs)	4 fl. oz.	280
Chocolate chip cookie (Good Humor)	1 sandwich	480
Chocolate eclair (Good Humor) bar	3-fl.-oz piece	180
Chocolate malt bar (Good Humor)	3-fl. oz. bar	190
Chocolate raspberry truffle (Baskin-Robbins)	4 fl. oz.	310
Coffee:		
(Breyers)	½ cup	140
(Häagen-Dazs) chip	4 fl. oz.	272
Cookies & cream:		
(Breyer's)	½ cup	170
(Häagen-Dazs)	4 fl. oz.	272
(Sealtest)	½ cup	150
Cookie sandwich (Good Humor)	2.7 fl. oz. piece	290
Eskimo Pie, vanilla with chocolate coating	3-fl.-oz. bar	180
Eskimo, Thin Mint, with chocolate coating	2-fl.-oz. bar	140
Fat Frog (Good Humor)	3-fl.-oz. pop	140
Fudge royal (Sealtest)	½ cup	140
Grand marnier (Baskin-Robbins)	4 fl. oz.	240
Heart (Good Humor)	4-fl.-oz. pop	200
Honey (Häagen-Dazs)	4 fl. oz.	256
Jamocha (Baskin-Robbins)	1 scoop (2½ fl. oz.)	146
Key lime & cream (Häagen-Dazs)	4 fl. oz.	192
Macadamia nut (Häagen-Dazs)	4 fl. oz.	320
Maple walnut (Häagen-Dazs)	4 fl. oz.	312
Mint chocolate chip (Breyers)	½ cup	170
Oreo, Cookies 'n Cream:		
Bulk	3 fl. oz.	140
Sandwich	1 piece	240
Peach (Häagen-Dazs)	4 fl. oz.	212
Pralines 'N Cream (Baskin-Robbins)	1 scoop (2½ fl. oz.)	177
Rocky Road (Baskin-Robbins)	4 fl. oz.	291
Rum raisin (Häagen-Dazs)	4 fl. oz.	240
Sandwich (Good Humor)	2½-oz. piece	170
Shark (Good Humor)	3-fl.-oz. pop	70
Strawberry:		
(Baskin-Robbins) wild, light	4 fl. oz.	90
(Breyers)	½ cup	130
(Häagen-Dazs)	4 fl. oz.	232
(Howard Johnson's)	½ cup	187
Toasted almond bar (Good Humor)	3-fl.-oz. piece	190
Vanilla:		
(Baskin-Robbins) regular	4 fl. oz.	235

Food and Description	Measure or Quantity	Calories
(Häagen-Dazs)	4 fl. oz.	250
(Howard Johnson's)	½ cup	210
(Meadow Gold)	½ cup	140
(Sealtest)	½ cup	140
Vanilla slice (Good Humor):		
Regular	3.2-fl.-oz. slice	110
Calorie controlled	3.2-fl.-oz. slice	60
Vanilla swiss almond		
(Häagen-Dazs)	4 fl. oz.	300
Whammy (Good Humor)		
assorted	1.6-oz. piece	90
ICE CREAM CONE, cone only		
(Comet) regular	1 piece	40
ICE CREAM CUP, cup only		
(Comet) regular	1 cup	20
***ICE CREAM MIX** (Salada)		
any flavor	1 cup	310
ICE MILK:		
Hardened	¼ pt.	100
Soft-serve	¼ pt.	133
(Dean) *Count Calorie*	¼ pt.	99
(Light 'n Lively) coffee	½ cup	100
(Meadow Gold) vanilla, 4% fat	¼ pt.	95
ITALIAN DINNER, frozen		
(Banquet)	12-oz. dinner	597

J

JACK IN THE BOX RESTAURANT:		
Breakfast Jack	4.4-oz. serving	307
Burger:		
Regular	3.6-oz. serving	288
Cheeseburger:		
Regular	4-oz. serving	325
Bacon	8.1-oz. serving	705
Ultimate	9.9-oz. serving	942
Ham & Swiss	9.1-oz. serving	754
Jumbo Jack:		
Regular	7.8-oz. serving	584
With cheese	8.5-oz. serving	677
Monterey Burger	9.9-oz. serving	865
Mushroom	6.4-oz. serving	470
Swiss & bacon	6.6-oz. serving	678
Canadian crescent	4.7-oz. serving	452
Cheesecake	3.5-oz. serving	309
Chicken strips	1 piece	87
Chicken supreme sandwich	8.1-oz. serving	575
Club pita sandwich, excluding sauce	6.3-oz. serving	277

Food and Description	Measure or Quantity	Calories
Coffee, black	8 fl. oz.	2
Dinner in the Box (excluding sauce):		
Chicken strip	11.3-oz. serving	689
Shrimp	10.6-oz. serving	731
Sirloin Steak	11.8-oz. serving	699
Egg, scrambled, platter	8.8-oz. serving	662
Egg roll	1 piece	135
Fish supreme sandwich	8-oz. sandwich	554
French fries:		
Regular	2.4-oz. order	221
Large	3.8-oz. order	353
Jumbo	4.8-oz. order	442
Hot chocolate	8 fl. oz.	133
Jelly, grape	.5-oz. serving	38
Ketchup	1 serving	10
Mayonnaise	1 serving	152
Milk, low fat	8 fl. oz.	122
Milk shake:		
Chocolate	11.4-oz. serving	330
Strawberry	11.4-oz. serving	320
Vanilla	11.2-oz. serving	320
Moby Jack sandwich	4.8-oz. sandwich	444
Mustard	1 serving	8
Nachos:		
Cheese	6-oz. serving	571
Supreme	11.9-oz. serving	787
Onion rings	3.8-oz. serving	382
Orange juice	6.5-oz. serving	80
Pancake platter	8.1-oz. serving	612
Pizza pocket sandwich	5.7-oz. serving	497
Salad:		
Chef	13-oz. salad	295
Pasta & seafood	14.7-oz. salad	394
Side	3.9-oz. salad	51
Taco	12.6-oz. salad	377
Salad dressing:		
Regular:		
Blue cheese	1.2-oz. serving	131
Buttermilk	1.2-oz. serving	181
Thousand Island	1.2-oz. serving	156
Dietetic or low calorie, French	1.2-oz. serving	80
Sauce:		
A-1	1.8-oz. serving	35
BBQ	.9-oz. serving	39
Guacamole	.9-oz. serving	55
Mayo-mustard	.8-oz. serving	124
Mayo-onion	.8-oz. serving	143
Salsa	.9-oz. serving	8
Seafood cocktail	1.8-oz. serving	57
Sweet & sour	1-oz. serving	40
Sausage crescent	5.5-oz. serving	585
Shrimp	1 piece (.3 oz.)	27

Food and Description	Measure or Quantity	Calories
Soft drink:		
Sweetened:		
Coca-Cola Classic	12 fl. oz.	144
Dr. Pepper	12 fl. oz.	144
Root beer, *Ramblin'*	12 fl. oz.	176
Sprite	12 fl. oz.	144
Diet, *Coca-Cola*	12 fl. oz.	Tr.
Supreme crescent	5.1-oz. serving	547
Syrup, pancake	1.5-oz. serving	121
Taco:		
Regular	2.9-oz. serving	191
Super	4.8-oz. serving	288
Tea, iced, plain	12 fl. oz.	3
Turnover, hot apple	4.2-oz. piece	410
JELL-O FRUIT BAR	1 bar	45
JELL-O FRUIT & CREAM BAR	1 bar	72
JELL-O GELATIN POPS:		
Cherry, grape or strawberry	1 pop	37
Raspberry	1 pop	34
JELL-O PUDDING POPS:		
Chocolate, chocolate with chocolate chips & vanilla with chocolate chips	1 bar	80
Chocolate covered chocolate & vanilla	1 bar	130
JELLY, sweetened (See also individual flavors)		
(Crosse & Blackwell) all flavors	1 T.	51
JERUSALEM ARTICHOKE, pared	4 oz.	75
JOHANNISBERG RIESLING WINE (Louis M. Martini)	3 fl. oz.	61

K

KABOOM, cereal (General Mills)	1 cup	110
KALE:		
Boiled, leaves only	4 oz.	110
Canned (Allen's) chopped, solids & liq.	½ cup	25
Frozen:		
(Birds Eye) chopped	⅓ pkg.	32
(McKenzie) chopped	3⅓ oz.	30
(Southland) chopped	⅕ of 16-oz. pkg.	25
KARO SYRUP (See SYRUP)		
KEFIR (Alta-Dena Dairy):		
Plain	1 cup	180
Flavored	1 cup	190
KIDNEY:		
Beef, braised	4 oz.	286
Calf, raw	4 oz.	128
Lamb, raw	4 oz.	119

Food and Description	Measure or Quantity	Calories
KIELBASA (see **SAUSAGE,** Polish-style)		
KING VITAMAN, cereal (Quaker)	1¼ cups	113
KIPPER SNACKS (King David Brand) Norwegian	3¼-oz. can	195
KIX, cereal	1½ cups	110
KNOCKWURST	1 oz.	79
*_KOOL-AID_ (General Foods):		
Unsweetened (sugar to be added)	8 fl. oz.	98
Pre-sweetened:		
Regular, sugar sweetened:		
Apple or sunshine punch	8 fl. oz.	96
Cherry or grape	8 fl. oz.	89
Tropical punch	8 fl. oz.	99
Dietetic, sugar-free:		
Cherry or grape	8 fl. oz.	2
Sunshine punch	8 fl. oz.	4
KUMQUAT, flesh & skin	5 oz.	74

L

Food and Description	Measure or Quantity	Calories
LAMB:		
Leg:		
Roasted, lean & fat	3 oz.	237
Roasted, lean only	3 oz.	158
Loin, one 5-oz. chop (weighed with bone before cooking) will give you:		
Lean & fat	2.8 oz.	280
Lean only	2.3 oz.	122
Rib, one 5-oz. chop (weighed with bone before cooking) will give you:		
Lean & fat	2.9 oz.	334
Lean only	2 oz.	118
Shoulder:		
Roasted, lean & fat	3 oz.	287
Roasted, lean only	3 oz.	174
LASAGNA:		
Canned (Hormel) _Short Orders_	7½-oz. can	260
Frozen:		
(Armour) _Dinner Classics_	10-oz. meal	380
(Celentano):		
Regular	½ of 16-oz. pkg.	320
Primavera	11-oz. pkg.	300
(Conagra) _Light & Elegant_	11¼-oz. entree	280
(Le Menu) vegetable	11-oz. dinner	360
(Stouffer's) _Lean Cuisine_	11-oz. meal	240

Food and Description	Measure or Quantity	Calories
(Swanson):		
Hungry Man, with meat	18¾-oz. dinner	730
Main Course, with meat	13¼-oz. entree	450
(Weight Watcher's) regular	12-oz. meal	360
LEEKS	4 oz.	59
LEMON:		
Whole	2⅛" lemon	22
Peeled	2⅛" lemon	20
LEMONADE:		
Canned:		
Capri Sun	6¾ fl. oz.	63
Country Time	6 fl. oz.	69
Chilled (Minute Maid) regular		
or pink	6 fl. oz.	79
*Frozen:		
Country Time, regular or pink	6 fl. oz.	68
Minute Maid	6 fl. oz.	74
*Mix:		
Regular:		
Country Time, regular or pink	6 fl. oz.	68
(Hi-C)	6 fl. oz.	76
Kool-Aid, sweetened, regular		
or pink	6 fl. oz.	65
Lemon Tree (Lipton)	6 fl. oz.	68
Dietetic:		
Crystal Light	8 fl. oz.	4
Kool-Aid	6 fl. oz.	3
(Sunkist)	8 fl. oz.	8
LEMONADE BAR (Sunkist)	3-fl.-oz. bar	70
LEMON EXTRACT (Virginia Dare)	1 tsp.	21
LEMON JUICE:		
Canned, *ReaLemon*	1 T.	3
*Frozen (Minute Maid) unsweetened	1 fl. oz.	77
***LEMON-LIMEADE DRINK**,		
Crystal Light	8 fl. oz.	4
LEMON PEEL, candied	1 oz.	90
LENTIL, cooked, drained	½ cup	107
LETTUCE:		
Bibb or Boston	4" head	23
Cos or Romaine, shredded or		
broken into pieces	½ cup	4
Grand Rapids, Salad Bowl		
or Simpson	2 large leaves	9
Iceberg, New York or Great Lakes	¼ of 4¾" head	15
LIFE, cereal (Quaker) regular or		
cinnamon	⅔ cup	105
LIL' ANGELS (Hostess)	1-oz. piece	90
LIME, peeled	2" dia.	15
***LIMEADE**, frozen (Minute Maid)	6 fl. oz.	75
LIME JUICE, *ReaLime*	1 T.	2
LINGUINI, frozen (Stouffer's)		
clam sauce	10½ oz.	285

Food and Description	Measure or Quantity	Calories
LIVER:		
Beef:		
Fried	6½″ × 2⅜″ × ⅜″ slice	195
Cooked (Swift)	3.2-oz. serving	141
Calf, fried	6½″ × 2⅛″ × ⅜″ slice	222
Chicken, simmered	2″ × 2″ × ⅝″ piece	41
LIVERWURST SPREAD (Hormel)	1-oz. serving	70
LOBSTER:		
Cooked, meat only	1 cup	138
Canned, meat only	4-oz. serving	108
Frozen, South African lobster tail		
3 in 8-oz. pkg.	1 piece	87
4 in 8-oz. pkg.	1 piece	65
5 in 8-oz. pkg.	1 piece	51
LOBSTER NEWBURG	1 cup	485
LOBSTER PASTE, canned	1-oz. serving	51
LOBSTER SALAD	4-oz. serving	125
LONG ISLAND TEA COCKTAIL		
(Mr. Boston) 12½% alcohol	3 fl. oz.	93
LONG JOHN SILVER'S:		
Catfish fillet	2.7-oz. piece	203
Catsup	.4 oz.	12
Chicken plank	1.4-oz. piece	104
Chicken sandwich	6.1-oz. sandwich	562
Chowder, clam	1 order	128
Clams, breaded	4.7-oz. order	526
Coleslaw	3½ oz. (drained on fork)	182
Corn on the cob	5.3-oz. ear	176
Cracker	1 piece	12
Drinks:		
Regular, carbonated or non-carbonated	10 fl. oz.	120
Dietetic	10 fl. oz.	Tr.
Fish fillet:		
Baked, with sauce	5.5-oz. serving	151
Batter fried	3-oz. piece	202
Kitchen breaded	2-oz. piece	122
Fish sandwich	6.4-oz. sandwich	555
Fryer	3-oz. serving	247
Hush puppies	.85-oz. piece	72
Oyster, breaded, fried	.7-oz. piece	60
Peg Leg, battered	1-oz. piece	91
Pie:		
Apple	4-oz. piece	280
Cherry	4-oz. piece	294
Lemon meringue	3½-oz. piece	200
Pecan	4-oz. piece	446
Pumpkin	4-oz. piece	251
Scallop, batter fried	.7-oz. piece	53
Seafood salad	5.8 oz. serving	386
Seafood sauce	1.2-oz. serving	34

Food and Description	Measure or Quantity	Calories
Shrimp:		
Batter fried	.6-oz. piece	47
Breaded, fried	4.7-oz. order	388
Chilled	.2-oz. piece	6
Tartar sauce	1-oz. serving	119
Vegetables, mixed	4-oz. serving	54
LOQUAT, fresh, flesh only	2 oz.	27
LUCKY CHARMS, cereal (General Mills)	1 cup	110
LUNCHEON MEAT (See also individual listings such as BOLOGNA, HAM, etc.):		
Banquet loaf (Eckrich)	¾-oz. slice	50
Bar-B-Que loaf (Oscar Mayer) 90% fat free	1-oz. slice	48
Beef, jellied loaf (Hormel)	1.2-oz. slice	45
Gourmet loaf (Eckrich)	1-oz. slice	35
Ham & cheese (See HAM & CHEESE)		
Ham roll sausage (Oscar Mayer)	1-oz. slice	43
Honey loaf:		
(Eckrich)	1-oz. slice	40
(Hormel)	1 slice	55
(Oscar Mayer)	1-oz. slice	35
Iowa brand (Hormel)	1 slice	45
Liver cheese (Oscar Mayer)	1.3-oz. slice	116
Liver loaf (Hormel)	1 slice	80
Macaroni-cheese loaf (Eckrich)	1-oz. slice	68
Meat loaf	1-oz. serving	57
New England brand sliced sausage:		
(Eckrich)	1-oz. slice	35
(Oscar Mayer) 92% fat free	.8-oz. slice	22
Old fashioned loaf (Oscar Mayer)	1-oz. slice	64
Olive loaf:		
(Eckrich)	1-oz. slice	80
(Hormel)	1-oz. slice	55
(Oscar Mayer)	1-oz. slice	62
Peppered loaf:		
(Eckrich)	1-oz. slice	40
(Hormel) Light & Lean	1 slice	50
(Oscar Mayer) 93% fat free	1-oz. slice	43
Pickle loaf:		
(Eckrich)	1-oz. slice	80
(Hormel)	1 slice	60
Pickle & pimiento (Oscar Mayer)	1-oz. slice	63
Pressed luncheon sausage (Oscar Mayer)	.8-oz. slice	35
Spiced (Hormel)	1 slice	75

M

Food and Description	Measure or Quantity	Calories
MACADAMIA NUT		
(Royal Hawaiian)	1 oz.	197
MACARONI:		
Cooked:		
8-10 minutes, firm	1 cup	192
14-20 minutes, tender	1 cup	155
Canned (Franco-American) *PizzOs*	7½-oz. can	170
Frozen:		
(Morton) & beef	10-oz. dinner	245
(Swanson) & beef	12-oz. dinner	360
MACARONI & CHEESE:		
Canned:		
(Franco-American) regular or elbow	7⅜-oz. serving	170
(Hormel) *Short Orders*	7½-oz. can	170
Frozen:		
(Banquet):		
Casserole	8-oz. pkg.	344
Dinner	9-oz. dinner	334
(Celentano) baked	½ of 12-oz. pkg.	290
(Conagra) *Light & Elegant*	9-oz. entree	300
(Morton)	20-oz. casserole	648
(Stouffer's)	6-oz. serving	260
(Swanson)	12¼-oz. dinner	380
Mix:		
(Golden Grain) deluxe	¼ pkg.	190
*(Kraft):		
Regular, plain	¼ box	190
Velveeta, shells	¼ box	270
*(Prince)	¾ cup	268
MACARONI & CHEESE PIE, frozen (Swanson)	7-oz. pie	210
MACARONI SALAD, canned (Nalley's)	4-oz. serving	206
MACKEREL, Atlantic, broiled with fat	8½″ × 2½″ × ½″ fillet	248
MAGIC SHELL (Smucker's)	1 T.	95
MALTED MILK MIX (Carnation):		
Chocolate	3 heaping tsps.	85
Natural	3 heaping tsps.	88
MALT LIQUOR, *Colt 45*	12 fl. oz.	156
MALT-O-MEAL, cereal	1 T.	33
MANDARIN ORANGE (See TANGERINE)		
MANGO, fresh	1 med. mango	88

Food and Description	Measure or Quantity	Calories
MANGO NECTAR (Libby's)	6 fl. oz.	60
MANHATTAN COCKTAIL		
(Mr. Boston) 20% alcohol	3 fl. oz.	123
MANICOTTI, frozen (Celentano):		
Without sauce	1 piece	85
With sauce	1 piece	150
MAPLE SYRUP (See SYRUP, Maple)		
MARGARINE:		
Regular:	1 pat (1″ × 1.3″ × 1″, 5 grams)	36
(Mazola)	1 T.	104
(Parkay) regular, soft or squeeze	1 T.	101
Imitation or dietetic:		
(Parkay)	1 T.	55
(Weight Watchers)	1 T.	50
Whipped		
(Blue Bonnet; Miracle; Parkay)	1 T.	67
MARGARITA COCKTAIL		
(Mr. Boston):		
Regular	3 fl. oz.	105
Strawberry	3 fl. oz.	138
MARINADE MIX:		
Chicken (Adolph's)	1-oz. packet	64
Meat:		
(French's)	1-oz. pkg.	80
(Kikkoman)	1-oz. pkg.	64
MARJORAM (French's)	1 tsp.	4
MARMALADE:		
Sweetened:		
(Keiller)	1 T.	60
(Smucker's)	1 T.	53
Dietetic:		
(Estee; Louis Sherry)	1 T.	6
(Featherweight)	1 T.	16
(S&W) *Nutradiet,* red label	1 T.	12
MARSHMALLOW FLUFF	1 heaping tsp.	59
MARSHMALLOW KRISPIES, cereal		
(Kellogg's)	1¼ cups	140
MARTINI COCKTAIL (Mr. Boston):		
Gin, extra dry, 20% alcohol	3 fl. oz.	99
Vodka, 20% alcohol	3 fl. oz.	102
MASA HARINA (Quaker)	⅓ cup	137
MASA TRIGO (Quaker)	⅓ cup	149
MATZO (Manischewitz):		
Regular:		
Plain	1-oz piece	110
Egg	1 cracker	108
Miniature	1 cracker	9
Tam Tam	1 cracker	15

Food and Description	Measure or Quantity	Calories
Wheat	1 cracker	9
Dietetic:		
Tam Tam, unsalted	1 cracker	14
Thins	.8 oz. piece	91
MATZO FARFEL		
(Manischewitz)	½ cup	143
MAYONNAISE:		
Real:		
Hellmann's (Best Foods)	1 T.	103
(Kraft)	1 T.	100
(Rokeach)	1 T.	100
Imitation or dietetic:		
(Estee)	1 T.	100
(Diet Delight) *Mayo-Lite*	1 T.	24
(Featherweight) *Soyamaise*	1 T.	100
(Kraft) light	1 T.	45
(Weight Watchers)	1 T.	40
MAYPO, cereal:		
30-second	¼ cup	89
Vermont style	¼ cup	121
McDONALD'S:		
Big Mac	1 hamburger	570
Biscuit:		
Plain	1 order	330
With bacon, egg & cheese	1 order	483
With sausage	1 order	467
With sausage & egg	1 order	585
Cheeseburger	1 cheeseburger	318
Chicken McNuggets	1 serving	323
Chicken McNuggets Sauce:		
Barbecue	1.1-oz. serving	60
Honey	.5-oz. serving	50
Hot mustard or sweet & sour	1.1-oz. serving	63
Cookies:		
Chocolate chip	1 package	342
McDonaldland	1 package	308
Egg McMuffin	1 serving	340
Egg, scrambled	1 serving	180
English muffin, with butter	1 muffin	186
Filet-O-Fish	1 sandwich	435
Grapefruit juice	6 fl. oz.	75
Hamburger	1 hamburger	263
Hot cakes with butter & syrup	1 serving	500
Pie:		
Apple	1 pie	253
Cherry	1 pie	260
Potato:		
Fried	1 regular order	220
Hash browns	1 order	125
Quarter Pounder:		
Regular	1 hamburger	427

Food and Description	Measure or Quantity	Calories
With cheese	1 hamburger	525
Chef's salad	1 serving	230
Garden salad	1 serving	110
Chicken oriental salad	1 serving	140
Shrimp salad	1 serving	105
Side salad	1 serving	55
Bacon bits	1 packet	15
Chow mein noodles	1 packet	45
Croutons	1 packet	50
Dressings:		
Blue cheese	1 packet	345
French	1 packet	230
House	1 packet	330
Oriental	1 packet	95
Thousand Island	1 packet	390
Lo-cal vinaigrette	1 packet	60
Sausage McMuffin:		
Plain	1 sandwich	427
With egg	1 sandwich	517
Sausage, pork	1 serving	210
Shake:		
Chocolate	1 serving	383
Strawberry	1 serving	362
Vanilla	1 serving	352
Sundae:		
Caramel	1 serving	361
Hot fudge	1 serving	357
Strawberry	1 serving	320
MEATBALL DINNER or ENTREE, frozen:		
(Green Giant) sweet & sour	9.9-oz. entree	370
(Swanson)	8¼-oz. entree	290
***MEATBALL SEASONING MIX**		
(Durkee) Italian style	1 cup	619
MEATBALL STEW:		
Canned *Dinty Moore* (Hormel)	7½-oz. serving	245
Frozen (Stouffer's) *Lean Cuisine*	10-oz. serving	240
MEATBALLS, SWEDISH, frozen:		
(Armour) *Dinner Classics*	11½-oz. meal	470
(Stouffer's) with noodles	11-oz. pkg.	475
MEAT LOAF DINNER, frozen:		
(Banquet):		
Dinner	11-oz. dinner	395
Entree for One	5-oz.	240
(Morton)	11-oz. dinner	371
(Swanson) with tomato sauce	9-oz. entree	310
MEAT LOAF SEASONING MIX:		
*(Bell's)	4½ oz.	300
(Contadina)	3¾-oz. pkg.	360
MEAT, POTTED:		
(Hormel)	1 T.	30
(Libby's)	1-oz. serving	55

Food and Description	Measure or Quantity	Calories
MEAT TENDERIZER:		
Regular (Adolph's; McCormick)	1 tsp.	2
Seasoned (McCormick)	1 tsp.	5
MELBA TOAST, salted (Old London):		
Garlic, onion or white rounds	1 piece	10
Pumpernickel, rye, wheat or white	1 piece	17
MELON BALL, in syrup, frozen	½ cup	72
MENUDO, canned (Hormel) *Casa Grande*	7½-oz. can	90
MERLOT WINE (Louis M. Martini) 12½% alcohol	3 fl. oz.	60
MEXICALI DOGS, frozen (Hormel)	5-oz. serving	400
MEXICAN DINNER, frozen:		
(Morton)	11-oz. dinner	300
(Swanson)	16-oz. dinner	580
(Van de Kamp's) combination	11½-oz. dinner	420
MILK BREAK BARS (Pillsbury):		
Chocolate or chocolate mint	1 bar	230
Natural	1 bar	220
MILK, CONDENSED, *Eagle Brand* (Borden)	1 T.	64
***MILK, DRY,** non-fat, instant (Alba; Carnation, Pet; *Sanalac*)	1 cup	80
MILK, EVAPORATED:		
Regular:		
(Carnation)	1 fl. oz.	42
(Pet)	1 fl. oz.	43
Filled (Pet)	½ cup	150
Low fat (Carnation)	1 fl. oz.	27
Skimmed, (Carnation; *Pet 99*)	1 fl. oz.	25
MILK, FRESH:		
Buttermilk (Friendship)	8 fl. oz.	120
Chocolate:		
(Hershey's)	8 fl. oz.	190
(Nestlé) *Quik*	8 fl. oz.	220
Low fat, *Viva*, 2% fat	8 fl. oz.	130
Skim (Dairylea; Meadow Gold)	1 cup	90
Whole:		
(Dairylea)	1 cup	150
(Meadow Gold)	1 cup	120
MILK, GOAT, whole	1 cup	163
MILK, HUMAN	1 cup	163
MILNOT, dairy vegetable blend	1 fl. oz.	38
MINERAL WATER (La Croix)	Any quantity	0
MINI-WHEATS, cereal (Kellogg's) frosted	1 biscuit	28
MINT LEAVES	½ oz.	4
MOLASSES:		
Barbados	1 T.	51
Blackstrap	1 T.	40
Dark (Brer Rabbit)	1 T.	33

Food and Description	Measure or Quantity	Calories
Light	1 T.	48
Medium	1 T.	44
Unsulphured (Grandma's)	1 T.	60
MORTADELLA sausage	1 oz.	89
MOST, cereal (Kellogg's)	½ cup	100
MOUSSE, canned, dietetic		
(Featherweight) chocolate	½ cup	100
MUFFIN:		
Apple (Pepperidge Farm) with spice	1 muffin	170
Blueberry:		
(Morton) rounds	1.5-oz. muffin	110
(Pepperidge Farm)	1.9-oz. muffin	180
Bran (Pepperidge Farm)	1 muffin	180
Carrot walnut (Pepperidge Farm)	1 muffin	170
Chocolate chip (Pepperidge Farm)	1 muffin	170
Corn:		
(Morton)	1.7-oz. muffin	130
(Pepperidge Farm)	1.9-oz. muffin	180
English:		
(Pepperidge Farm):		
Plain	2-oz. muffin	140
Cinnamon, raisin	2-oz. muffin	150
Roman Meal	2.3-oz. muffin	150
(Thomas'):		
Regular or frozen or sour-dough	2-oz. muffin	133
Raisin	2.2-oz. muffin	153
(Wonder)	2-oz. muffin	130
Plain	1.4-oz. muffin	118
Sourdough (Wonder)	2-oz. muffin	130
MUFFIN MIX:		
Blueberry:		
*(Betty Crocker) wild	1 muffin	120
(Duncan Hines)	1/12 pkg.	99
Bran:		
(Duncan Hines)	1/12 pkg.	97
(Elam's) natural	1 T.	23
*Cherry (Betty Crocker)	1/12 pkg.	120
Corn:		
*(Betty Crocker)	1 muffin	160
*(Dromedary)	1 muffin	120
MULLIGAN STEW, canned, *Dinty Moore, Short Orders* (Hormel)	7½-oz. can	230
MUSCATEL WINE (Gallo)		
14% alcohol	3 fl. oz.	86
MUSHROOM:		
Raw, whole	½ lb.	62
Raw, trimmed, sliced	½ cup	10
Canned (Green Giant) solids & liq., whole or sliced:		
Regular	2-oz. serving	14

Food and Description	Measure or Quantity	Calories
B & B	1½-oz. serving	18
MUSHROOM, CHINESE, dried	1 oz.	81
MUSSEL, in shell	1 lb.	153
MUSTARD:		
Powder (French's)	1 tsp.	9
Prepared:		
Brown (French's; Gulden's)	1 tsp.	5
Chinese (Chun King)	1 tsp.	5
Dijon, *Grey Poupon*	1 tsp.	6
Horseradish (Nalley's)	1 tsp.	5
Yellow (Gulden's)	1 tsp.	5
MUSTARD GREENS:		
Canned (Allens) solids & liq.	½ cup	20
Frozen:		
(Birds Eye)	⅓ pkg.	25
(Frosty Acres)	3.3 oz.	20
(Southland)	⅓ of 16-oz. pkg.	20
MUSTARD SPINACH:		
Raw	1 lb.	100
Boiled, drained, no added salt	4-oz. serving	18

N

NATHAN'S:		
French fries	Regular order	550
Hamburger	1 sandwich	360
Hot dog & roll	1 order	290
NATURAL CEREAL:		
Familia:		
Regular	½ cup	187
Bran	½ cup	166
No added sugar	½ cup	181
Heartland:		
Plain, coconut or raisin	¼ cup	130
Trail mix	¼ cup	120
(Quaker):		
Hot, whole wheat	⅓ cup	106
100%	¼ cup	138
100% with raisins & dates	¼ cup	134
NATURE SNACKS (Sun-Maid):		
Carob Crunch	1 oz.	143
Carob Peanut	1¼ oz.	190
Carob Raisin or Yogurt Raisin	1¼ oz.	160
Tahitian Treat or Yogurt Crunch	1 oz.	123
NECTARINE, flesh only	4 oz.	73
NOODLE:		
Cooked, 1½″ strips	1 cup	200
Dry (Pennsylvania Dutch Brand)		
broad	1 oz.	105

Food and Description	Measure or Quantity	Calories
NOODLE, CHOW MEIN:		
(Chun King)	1 oz.	139
(La Choy)	½ cup (1 oz.)	150
NOODLE MIX:		
*(Betty Crocker):		
Fettucini Alfredo	¼ pkg.	220
Stroganoff	¼ pkg.	240
*(Lipton) & sauce:		
Regular:		
Beef, butter, chicken or sour		
cream & chive	½ cup	190
Cheese	½ cup	200
Deluxe:		
Alfredo	½ cup	220
Chicken bombay	½ cup	190
Stroganoff	½ cup	200
NOODLE, RICE (La Choy)	1 oz.	130
NOODLE ROMANOFF, frozen		
(Stouffer's)	⅓ pkg.	170
NOODLES & BEEF:		
Canned (Hormel) *Short Orders*	7½-oz. can	230
Frozen (Banquet) *Buffet Supper*	2-lb. pkg.	754
NOODLES & CHICKEN:		
Canned (Hormel) *Dinty Moore,*		
Short Orders	7½-oz. can	210
Frozen (Swanson)	10½-oz. dinner	270
NUT (See specific type: CASHEW, MACADAMIA, etc.)		
NUT, MIXED:		
Dry roasted:		
(Flavor House)	1 oz.	172
(Planters) salted	1 oz.	160
Oil roasted (Planters) with or without		
peanuts	1 oz.	180
NUTMEG (French's)	1 tsp.	11
NUTRI-GRAIN, cereal (Kellogg's):		
Corn	½ cup	110
Wheat	⅔ cup	110
Wheat & Raisin	⅔ cup	140
NUTRIMATO (Mott's)	6 fl. oz.	70

O

OAT FLAKES, cereal (Post)	⅔ cup	107
OATMEAL:		
Dry:		
Regular:		
(Elam's) Scotch style	1 oz.	108
(H-O) old fashioned	1 T.	15

Food and Description	Measure or Quantity	Calories
(3-Minute Brand)	⅓ cup	110
Instant:		
(H-O):		
Regular, boxed	1 T.	15
With bran & spice	1½-oz. packet	157
With maple & brown sugar flavor	1½-oz. packet	160
(Quaker):		
Regular	1-oz. packet	105
Apple & cinnamon	1¼-oz. packet	134
Raisins & spice	1½-oz. packet	159
(3-Minute Brand)	½-oz. packet	162
Quick:		
(Harvest Brand)	⅓ cup	108
(Ralston Purina)	⅓ cup	110
(3-Minute Brand)	⅓ cup	110
Cooked, regular	1 cup	132
OIL, SALAD OR COOKING:		
(Bertoli) olive	1 T.	120
Crisco, Mazola	1 T.	126
Mrs. Tucker's; (Goya)	1 T.	130
Sunlite: Wesson	1 T.	120
OKRA, frozen:		
(Birds Eye) whole, baby	⅓ pkg.	36
(Frosty Acres):		
Cut	3.3 oz.	25
White	3.3 oz.	30
(Seabrook Farms) cut	⅓ pkg.	32
(Southland) cut	⅕ of 16-oz. pkg.	30
OLD FASHIONED COCKTAIL		
(Hiram Walker) 62 proof	3 fl. oz.	165
OLIVE:		
Green	4 med. or 3 extra large or 2 giant	19
Ripe, Mission	3 small or 2 large	18
OMELET, frozen (Swanson)		
TV Brand, Spanish style	7¾-oz. entree	240
ONION:		
Raw	2½" onion	38
Boiled, pearl onion	½ cup	27
Canned (Durkee) *O & C:*		
Boiled	¼ of 16-oz. jar.	32
Creamed	¼ of 15½-oz. can	554
Dehydrated (Gilroy) flakes	1 tsp.	5
Frozen:		
(Birds Eye):		
Creamed	⅓ pkg.	106
Whole, small	⅓ pkg.	44
(Frosty Acres) chopped	1 oz.	8
(Green Giant) in cheese sauce	½ cup	90
(Mrs. Paul's) french-fried rings	½ of 5-oz. pkg.	167
ONION BOUILLON:		

Food and Description	Measure or Quantity	Calories
(Herb-Ox)	1 cube	10
MBT	1 packet	16
ONION, COCKTAIL		
(Vlasic)	1 oz.	4
ONION, GREEN	1 small onion	4
ONION SALAD SEASONING		
(French's) instant	1 T.	15
ONION SALT (French's)	1 tsp.	6
ONION SOUP (See SOUP, Onion)		
ORANGE:		
Peeled	½ cup	62
Sections	4 oz.	58
ORANGE-APRICOT JUICE		
COCKTAIL, *Musselman's*	8 fl. oz.	100
ORANGE DRINK:		
Canned:		
Capri Sun	6¾-fl.-oz. can	103
(Hi-C)	8 fl. oz.	123
(Lincoln)	6 fl. oz.	90
*Mix:		
Regular (Hi-C)	8 fl. oz.	91
Dietetic:		
Crystal Light	6 fl. oz.	4
(Sunkist)	6 fl. oz.	6
ORANGE EXTRACT (Durkee)		
imitation	1 tsp.	15
ORANGE-GRAPEFRUIT JUICE:		
Canned (Libby's) unsweetened	6 fl. oz.	80
*Frozen (Minute Maid) unsweetened	6 fl. oz.	76
ORANGE JUICE:		
Canned:		
(Del Monte) unsweetened	6 fl. oz.	80
(Libby's) unsweetened	6 fl. oz.	90
(Texsun) sweetened	6 fl. oz.	83
Chilled (Sunkist)	6 fl. oz.	80
*Frozen:		
(Birds Eye) *Orange Plus*	6 fl. oz.	95
Bright & Early, imitation	6 fl. oz.	90
(Sunkist)	6 fl. oz.	80
ORANGE JUICE BAR (Sunkist)	3-fl.-oz. bar	70
ORANGE JUICE DRINK, canned		
(Sunkist)	8.45 fl. oz.	140
ORANGE PEEL, CANDIED	1 oz.	93
ORANGE-PINEAPPLE DRINK,		
canned (Lincoln)	6 fl. oz.	90
ORANGE-PINEAPPLE JUICE,		
canned (Texsun)	8 fl. oz.	89
ORCHARD BLEND JUICE,		
canned (Welch's):		
Apple-grape	6 fl. oz.	100
Harvest	6 fl. oz.	90
Vineyard	6 fl. oz.	120

Food and Description	Measure or Quantity	Calories
OVALTINE, chocolate	¾ oz.	78
OVEN FRY (General Foods):		
Crispy crumb for pork	4.2-oz. envelope	484
Crispy crumb for chicken	4.2-oz. envelope	460
Homestyle flour recipe	3.2-oz. envelope	304
OYSTER:		
Raw:		
Eastern	19–31 small or 13–19 med.	158
Pacific & Western	6–9 small or 4–6 med.	218
Canned (Bumble Bee) shelled, whole, solids & liq.	1 cup	218
Fried	4 oz.	271
OYSTER STEW, home recipe	½ cup	103

P

Food and Description	Measure or Quantity	Calories
PAC-MAN, cereal (General Mills)	1 cup	110
***PANCAKE BATTER**, frozen (Aunt Jemima):		
Plain	4" pancake	70
Blueberry or buttermilk	4" pancake	68
PANCAKE DINNER OR ENTREE, frozen (Swanson):		
& blueberry sauce	7-oz. meal	400
& sausage	6-oz. meal	460
PANCAKE & SAUSAGE, frozen (Swanson)	6-oz. entree	440
***PANCAKE & WAFFLE MIX:**		
Plain:		
(Aunt Jemima) Original	4" pancake	73
(Log Cabin) Complete	4" pancake	58
(Pillsbury) *Hungry Jack:*		
Complete, bulk	4" pancake	63
Extra Lights	4" pancake	70
Golden Blend, complete	4" pancake	80
Panshakes	4" pancake	83
Blueberry (Pillsbury) *Hungry Jack*	4" pancake	107
Buckwheat (Aunt Jemima)	4" pancake	67
Buttermilk:		
(Aunt Jemima) regular	4" pancake	100
(Betty Crocker) complete	4" pancake	70
(Pillsbury) *Hungry Jack*, complete	4" pancake	63
Whole wheat (Aunt Jemima)	4" pancake	83
Dietetic:		
(Estee)	3" pancake	33
(Featherweight)	4" pancake	43
PANCAKE & WAFFLE SYRUP (See SYRUP, Pancake & Waffle)		

Food and Description	Measure or Quantity	Calories
PAPAYA, fresh:		
Cubed	½ cup	36
Juice	4 oz.	78
PAPRIKA (French's)	1 tsp.	7
PARSLEY:		
Fresh, chopped	1 T.	2
Dried (French's)	1 tsp.	4
PASSION FRUIT, giant, whole	1 lb.	53
PASTINAS, egg	1 oz.	109
PASTRAMI (Carl Buddig)	1 oz.	40
PASTRY SHEET, PUFF, frozen		
(Pepperidge Farm)	1 sheet	1150
PÂTE:		
De foie gras	1 T.	69
Liver:		
(Hormel)	1 T.	35
(Sell's)	1 T.	93
PDQ:		
Chocolate	1 T.	66
Strawberry	1 T.	60
PEA, green:		
Boiled	½ cup	58
Canned, regular pack, solids & liq.:		
(Comstock)	½ cup	70
(Del Monte) seasoned or sweet,		
regular size	½ cup	60
(Green Giant):		
Early with onions, sweet or		
sweet with onions	¼ of 17-oz. can	60
Sweet, mini	¼ of 17-oz. can	64
(Larsen) *Fresh-Lite*	½ cup	50
Canned, dietetic pack, solids & liq.:		
(Del Monte) no salt added,		
sweet	½ cup	60
(Diet Delight)	½ cup	50
(Featherweight) sweet	½ cup	70
(Larsen) *Fresh-Lite*, low sodium	½ cup	50
Frozen:		
(Birds Eye):		
Regular	⅓ pkg.	78
In butter sauce	⅓ pkg.	85
In cream sauce	⅓ pkg.	84
(Frosty Acres):		
Regular	3.3 oz.	80
Tiny	3.3 oz.	60
(Green Giant):		
In cream sauce	½ cup	100
Sweet, *Harvest Fresh*	½ cup	80
PEA & CARROT:		
Canned, regular pack, solids & liq.:		
(Comstock)	½ cup	60
(Del Monte)	½ cup	50

Food and Description	Measure or Quantity	Calories
(Libby's)	½ cup	56
Canned, dietetic pack, solids & liq.:		
(Diet Delight)	½ cup	40
(Larsen) *Fresh-Lite*, low sodium	½ cup	50
(S&W) *Nutradiet*	½ cup	35
Frozen:		
(Birds Eye)	⅓ pkg.	61
(McKenzie)	3.3-oz. serving	60
PEA, CROWDER, frozen		
(Southland)	⅕ of 16-oz. pkg.	130
PEA POD:		
Boiled, drained solids	4 oz.	49
Frozen (La Choy)	6-oz. pkg.	70
PEACH:		
Fresh, with thin skin	2″ dia.	38
Fresh slices	½ cup	32
Canned, regular pack, solids & liq.:		
(Del Monte) Cling:		
Halves or slices	½ cup	80
Spiced	3½ oz.	80
(Libby's) heavy syrup:		
Halves	½ cup	105
Sliced	½ cup	102
Canned, dietetic pack, solids & liq.:		
(Del Monte) Lite, Cling	½ cup	50
(Diet Delight) Cling:		
Juice pack	½ cup	50
Water Pack	½ cup	30
(Featherweight);		
Cling or Freestone, juice pack	½ cup	50
Cling, water pack	½ cup	30
(S&W) *Nutradiet,* Cling:		
Juice pack	½ cup	60
Water pack	½ cup	30
Frozen (Birds Eye)	5-oz. pkg.	141
PEACH BUTTER (Smucker's)	1 T.	45
PEACH DRINK, canned (Hi-C):		
Canned	6 fl.oz.	90
*Mix	6 fl. oz.	72
PEACH LIQUEUR (DeKuyper)	1 fl. oz.	82
PEACH NECTAR, canned (Libby's)	6 fl. oz.	90
PEACH PRESERVE OR JAM:		
Sweetened (Smucker's)	1 T.	53
Dietetic (Dia-Mel)	1 T.	6
PEANUT:		
In shell (Planters)	1 oz.	160
Dry roasted:		
(Fisher)	1 oz.	163
(Planters)	1 oz.	160
(Tom's)	1 oz.	160
Oil roasted (Planters) salted	1 oz.	170

Food and Description	Measure or Quantity	Calories
PEANUT BUTTER:		
Regular:		
(Adams)	1 T.	95
(Elam's) natural	1 T.	109
(Holsum)	1 T.	94
(Jif) creamy	1 T.	93
(Laura Scudder's)	1 T.	95
(Peter Pan):		
Crunchy	1 T.	101
Smooth	1 T.	94
(Skippy) creamy or super chunk	1 T.	108
Dietetic:		
(Adams) low sodium	1 T.	95
(S&W) *Nutradiet*, low sodium	1 T.	93
(Smucker's) low sodium	1 T.	100
PEANUT BUTTER BAKING		
CHIPS (Reese's)	3 T. (1 oz.)	153
PEAR:		
Whole	3″ × 2½″ pear	101
Canned, regular pack, solids & liq.:		
(Del Monte) Bartlett	½ cup	80
(Libby's)	½ cup	102
Canned, dietetic pack, solids & liq.:		
(Del Monte) Lite	½ cup	50
(Featherweight) Bartlett:		
Juice pack	½ cup	60
Water pack	½ cup	40
(Libby's) water pack	½ cup	60
Dried (Sun-Maid)	½ cup	260
PEAR-APPLE JUICE (Tree Top)	6 fl. oz.	90
PEAR-GRAPE JUICE (Tree Top)	6 fl. oz.	100
PEAR NECTAR, canned (Libby's)	6 fl. oz.	100
PEAR-PASSION FRUIT NECTAR,		
canned (Libby's)	6 fl. oz.	60
PEAR, STRAINED		
(Larsen)	½ cup	65
PEBBLES, cereal:		
Cocoa	⅞ cup	117
Fruity	⅞ cup	116
PECAN:		
Halves	6-7 pieces	48
Roasted, dry:		
(Fisher) salted	1 oz.	220
(Planters)	1 oz.	190
PECTIN, FRUIT:		
Certo	6-oz. pkg.	19
Sure-Jell	1¾-oz. pkg.	170
PEPPER:		
Black (French's)	1 tsp.	9
Seasoned (French's)	1 tsp.	8
PEPPER & ONION, frozen		
(Southland)	2-oz. serving	15

Food and Description	Measure or Quantity	Calories
PEPPER, BANANA (Vlasic)		
hot rings	1 oz.	4
PEPPER, CHERRY (Vlasic) mild	1 oz.	8
PEPPER, CHILI, canned:		
(Del Monte):		
Green, whole	½ cup	20
Jalapeño or chili, whole	½ cup	30
Old El Paso, green, chopped		
or whole	1 oz.	7
(Ortega):		
Diced, strips or whole	1 oz.	10
Jalapeño, diced or whole	1 oz.	9
(Vlasic) Jalapeño	1 oz.	8
PEPPERMINT EXTRACT (Durkee)		
imitation	1 tsp.	15
PEPPERONCINI (Vlasic)		
Greek, mild	1 oz.	4
PEPPERONI:		
(Eckrich)	1-oz. serving	135
(Hormel) regular or Rosa Grande	1-oz. serving	140
PEPPER STEAK, frozen:		
(Blue Star) *Dining Lite,* with rice	9½-oz. entree	267
(Le Menu)	11½-oz. dinner	360
(Stouffer's)	5¼-oz. serving	354
PEPPER, STUFFED:		
Home recipe	2¾″ × 2½″ pepper with 1⅛ cups stuffing	314
Frozen:		
(Celentano)	12½-oz. pkg.	290
(Stouffer's) green	7¾-oz. serving	225
(Weight Watchers) with veal stuffing	11¾-oz. meal	270
PEPPER, SWEET:		
Raw:		
Green:		
Whole	1 lb.	82
Without stem & seeds	1 med. pepper (2.6 oz.)	13
Red:		
Whole	1 lb.	112
Without stem & seeds	1 med. pepper (2.2 oz.)	19
Boiled, green, without salt, drained	1 med. pepper (2.6 oz.)	13
Frozen:		
(Frosty Acres) diced:		
Green	1 oz.	6
Red & green	1 oz.	7
(McKenzie)	1-oz. serving	6
(Southland) diced	2-oz. serving	10
PERCH, OCEAN:		
Atlantic, raw:		
Whole	1 lb.	124

Food and Description	Measure or Quantity	Calories
Meat only	4 oz.	108
Pacific, raw, whole	1 lb.	116
Frozen:		
(Banquet)	8¾-oz. dinner	434
(Mrs. Paul's) fillet, breaded & fried	2-oz. piece	145
(Van de Kamp's) batter dipped, french fried	2-oz. piece	135
PERNOD (Julius Wile)	1 fl. oz.	79
PERSIMMON:		
Japanese or Kaki, fresh:		
With seeds	4.4-oz. piece	79
Seedless	4.4-oz. piece	81
Native, fresh, flesh only	4-oz. serving	144
PHEASANT, raw, meat only	4-oz. serving	184
PICKLE:		
Cucumber, fresh or bread & butter:		
(Fannings)	1.2-oz. serving	17
(Featherweight) low sodium	1-oz. pickle	12
(Vlasic):		
Chips	1 oz.	7
Stix, sweet butter	1 oz.	5
Dill:		
(Featherweight) low sodium, whole	1-oz. serving	4
(Smucker's):		
Hamburger, sliced	1 slice	Tr.
Polish, whole	3½" pickle	8
(Vlasic):		
Original	1 oz.	2
No garlic	1 oz.	4
Hamburger (Vlasic) chips	1-oz. serving	2
Hot & spicy (Vlasic) garden mix	1 oz.	4
Kosher dill:		
(Claussen) halves or whole	2-oz. serving	7
(Featherweight) low sodium	1-oz. serving	4
(Smucker's):		
Baby	2¾"-long pickle	4
Whole	3½"-long pickle	8
(Vlasic)	1 oz.	4
Sweet:		
(Nalley's) *Nubbins*	1-oz. serving	28
(Smucker's):		
Gherkins	2"-long pickle	15
Whole	2½"-long pickle	18
(Vlasic)	1 oz.	30
Sweet & sour (Claussen) slices	1 slice	3
PIE:		
Regular, non-frozen:		
Apple:		
Home recipe, two crust	⅙ of 9" pie	404
(Hostess)	4½-oz. pie	390

Food and Description	Measure or Quantity	Calories
Banana, home recipe, cream or custard	⅙ of 9″ pie	336
Berry (Hostess)	4½-oz. pie	404
Blackberry, home recipe, two-crust	⅙ of 9″ pie	384
Blueberry:		
Home recipe, two-crust	⅙ of 9″ pie	382
(Hostess)	4½-oz. pie	394
Boston cream, home recipe	¹⁄₁₂ of 8″ pie	208
Butterscotch, home recipe, one-crust	⅙ of 9″ pie	406
Cherry:		
Home recipe, two-crust	⅙ of 9″ pie	412
(Hostess)	4½-oz. pie	390
Chocolate chiffon, home recipe	⅙ of 9″ pie	459
Chocolate meringue, home recipe	⅙ of 9″pie	353
Coconut custard, home recipe	⅙ of 9″pie	357
Lemon (Hostess)	4½-oz. pie	400
Lemon meringue, home recipe, one-crust	⅙ of 9″ pie	357
Mince, home recipe, two-crust	⅙ of 9″ pie	428
Peach (Hostess)	4½-oz. pie	400
Pumpkin, home recipe, one-crust	⅙ of 9″ pie	321
Raisin, home recipe, two-crust	⅙ of 9″ pie	427
Strawberry (Hostess)	4½-oz. pie	340
Frozen:		
Apple:		
(Banquet) family size	⅙ of 20-oz. pie	253
(Morton):		
Regular	⅙ of 24-oz. pie	296
Great Little Desserts, regular	8-oz. pie	590
(Weight Watchers)	3 oz.	180
Banana cream:		
(Banquet)	⅙ of 14-oz. pie	172
(Morton) regular	⅙ of 16-oz. pie	174
Blackberry (Banquet)	⅙ of 20-oz. pie	268
Blueberry:		
(Banquet)	⅙ of 20-oz. pie	266
(Morton) *Great Little Desserts*	8-oz. pie	580
Cherry:		
(Banquet)	⅙ of 20-oz. pie	252
(Morton) regular	⅙ of 24-oz. pie	300
(Weight Watchers)	3 oz.	200
Chocolate (Morton)	⅙ of 14-oz. pie	180
Chocolate cream:		
(Banquet)	⅙ of 14-oz. pie	177
(Morton) *Great Little Desserts*	3½-oz. pie	270
Coconut cream (Banquet)	⅙ of 14-oz. pie	179
Coconut custard (Morton) *Great Little Desserts*	6½-oz. pie	370
Lemon cream:		
(Banquet)	⅙ of 14-oz. pie	168

Food and Description	Measure or Quantity	Calories
(Morton) *Great Little Desserts*	3½-oz. pie	250
Mince:		
(Banquet)	⅙ of 20-oz. pie	258
(Morton)	⅙ of 24-oz. pie	310
Peach (Sara Lee)	⅙ of 31-oz. pie	458
Pumpkin:		
(Banquet)	⅙ of 20-oz. pie	197
(Morton) regular	⅙ of 24-oz. pie	230
Strawberry cream (Banquet)	⅙ of 14-oz. pie	168
PIECRUST:		
Home recipe, 9″ pie	1 crust	900
Refrigerated (Pillsbury)	2 crusts	1920
***PIECRUST MIX:**		
(Betty Crocker):		
Regular	¹⁄₁₆ pkg.	120
Stick	⅛ stick	120
(Flako)	⅙ of 9″ pie shell	245
(Pillsbury) mix or stick	⅙ of 2-crust pie	270
PIE FILLING (See also PUDDING OR PIE FILLING):		
Apple:		
(Comstock)	⅙ of 21-oz. can	110
(Thank You Brand)	3½ oz.	91
Apple rings or slices (See APPLE, canned)		
Apricot (Comstock)	⅙ of 21-oz. can	110
Banana cream (Comstock)	⅙ of 21-oz. can	110
Blueberry (Comstock)	⅙ of 21-oz. can	120
Cherry (Thank You Brand) regular	3½ oz.	99
Coconut cream (Comstock)	⅙ of 21-oz. can	120
Coconut custard, home recipe, made with egg yolk & milk	5 oz. (inc. crust)	288
Lemon (Comstock)	⅙ of 21-oz. can	160
Mincemeat (Comstock)	½ of 21-oz. can	170
Pumpkin (Libby's) (See also PUMPKIN, canned)	1 cup	210
Raisin (Comstock)	⅙ of 21-oz. can	140
***PIE MIX:**		
Boston Cream (Betty Crocker)	⅛ of pie	260
Chocolate (Royal)	⅛ of pie	260
PIEROGIES, frozen (Mrs. Paul's) potato & cheese	1 pierogi	90
PIGS FEET, pickled	4-oz. serving	226
PIMIENTO, canned:		
(Dromedary) drained	1-oz. serving	10
(Ortega)	¼ cup	6
(Sunshine) diced or sliced	1 T.	4
PIÑA COLADA (Mr. Boston) 12½% alcohol	3 fl. oz.	249
***PIÑA COLADA MIX** (Bar-Tender's)	5 fl. oz.	254

Food and Description	Measure or Quantity	Calories
PINEAPPLE:		
Fresh, chunks	½ cup	52
Canned, regular pack, solids & liq.:		
(Del Monte) slices, syrup pack	½ cup	90
(Dole):		
Juice pack, chunk, crushed or sliced	½ cup	70
Heavy syrup, chunk, crushed or sliced	½ cup	95
Canned, unsweetened or dietetic, solids & liq.:		
(Diet Delight) juice pack	½ cup	70
(Libby's) Lite	½ cup	60
(S&W) *Nutradiet*	1 slice	30
PINEAPPLE & GRAPEFRUIT JUICE DRINK, canned:		
(Del Monte) regular or pink	6 fl. oz.	90
(Dole) pink	6 fl. oz.	101
(Texsun)	6 fl. oz.	91
PINEAPPLE, CANDIED	1-oz. serving	90
PINEAPPLE FLAVORING (Durkee) imitation	1 tsp.	6
PINEAPPLE JUICE:		
Canned:		
(Del Monte)	6 fl. oz.	100
(Dole)	6 fl. oz.	103
(Texsun)	6 fl. oz.	97
*Frozen (Minute Maid)	6 fl. oz.	92
PINEAPPLE-ORANGE DRINK, canned (Hi-C)	6 fl. oz.	94
PINEAPPLE-ORANGE JUICE:		
Canned (Del Monte)	6 fl. oz.	90
*Frozen (Minute Maid)	6 fl. oz.	94
PINE NUT, pignolias, shelled	1 oz.	156
PINOT CHARDONNAY WINE (Paul Masson) 12% alcohol	3 fl. oz.	71
PISTACHIO NUT:		
In shell	½ cup	197
Shelled	¼ cup	184
(Fisher) shelled, roasted, salted	1 oz.	174
PIZZA PIE (See also **SHAKEY'S**):		
Regular, non-frozen:		
Home recipe	⅛ of 14″ pie	177
(*Domino's*):		
Beef, ground:		
Plain:		
12″ pizza (small)	1 slice	216
16″ pizza (large)	1 slice	303
With pepperoni:		
12″ pizza (small)	1 slice	216
16″ pizza (large)	1 slice	303

Food and Description	Measure or Quantity	Calories
Cheese:		
Plain:		
12" pizza (small)	1 slice	157
16" pizza (large)	1 slice	239
Double cheese:		
12" pizza (small)	1 slice	240
16" pizza (large)	1 slice	350
Double, with pepperoni		
12" pizza (small)	1 slice	227
16" pizza (large)	1 slice	389
Mushroom & sausage:		
12" pizza (small)	1 slice	183
16" pizza (large)	1 slice	266
Pepperoni:		
Plain:		
12" pizza (small)	1 slice	192
16" pizza (large)	1 slice	278
With mushrooms:		
12" pizza (small)	1 slice	194
16" pizza (large)	1 slice	280
With sausage:		
12" pizza (small)	1 slice	215
16" pizza (large)	1 slice	303
Sausage:		
12" pizza (small)	1 slice	180
16" pizza (large)	1 slice	264
Frozen:		
Canadian style bacon (Celeste)	8-oz. pie	483
Cheese:		
(Celentano):		
Mini slice	1 slice	157
Thick crust	⅓ of 13-oz. pie	238
(Stouffer's) French Bread	½ of 10⅜-oz. pkg.	330
(Weight Watchers)	6-oz. pie	350
Combination:		
(Celeste) Chicago style	¼ of 24-oz. pie	360
(La Pizzeria)	½ of 13½-oz. pie	420
(Van de Kamp's) thick crust	¼ of 24½-oz. pie	310
(Weight Watchers)	7¼-oz. pie	322
Deluxe:		
(Celeste)	½ of 9-oz. pie	281
(Stouffer's) French Bread	½ of 12⅜-oz. pkg.	400
Hamburger (Stouffer's) French Bread	½ of 12¼-oz. pkg.	400
Mushroom (Stouffer's) French Bread	½ of 12-oz. pkg.	340
Pepperoni:		
(Stouffer's) French Bread	½ of 11¼-oz. pkg.	410
(Weight Watchers)	6¼-oz. pie	370
Sausage:		
(Celeste)	½ of 8-oz. pie	262

Food and Description	Measure or Quantity	Calories
(Stouffer's) French Bread	½ of 12-oz. pkg.	420
(Weight Watchers) veal	6¾-oz. pie	350
Sausage & mushroom:		
(Celeste)	¼ of 24-oz. pie	365
(Stouffer's) French Bread	½ of 12½-oz. pkg.	395
Sicilian style (Celeste) deluxe	¼ of 26-oz. pie	408
Supreme (Celeste) without meat	½ of 8-oz. pie	217
*Mix (Ragú) *Pizza Quick*	¼ of pie	300
PIZZA SAUCE:		
(Contadina):		
Regular or with cheese	½ cup	80
With pepperoni	½ cup	90
(Ragú):		
Regular	2 oz.	32
Pizza Quick	2 oz.	45
PLUM:		
Fresh, Japanese & hybrid	2″ dia.	27
Fresh, prune-type, halves	½ cup	60
Canned, regular pack:		
(Stokely-Van Camp)	½ cup	120
(Thank You Brand) heavy syrup	½ cup	109
Canned, unsweetened, purple, solids & liq.:		
(Diet Delight) juice pack	½ cup	70
(Featherweight) water pack	½ cup	40
(S&W) *Nutradiet,* juice pack	½ cup	80
PLUM PRESERVE OR JAM, sweetened (Smucker's)	1 T.	53
PLUM PUDDING (Richardson & Robbins)	2″ wedge	270
POLYNESIAN-STYLE DINNER, frozen (Swanson)	12-oz. dinner	360
POMEGRANATE, whole	1 lb.	160
PONDEROSA RESTAURANT:		
A-1 Sauce	1 tsp.	4
Beef, chopped (patty only):		
Regular	3½ oz.	209
Double Deluxe	5.9 oz.	362
Junior (*Square Shooter*)	1.6 oz.	98
Steakhouse Deluxe	2.96 oz.	181
Beverages:		
Coca-Cola	8 fl. oz.	96
Coffee	6 fl. oz.	2
Dr. Pepper	8 fl. oz.	96
Milk, chocolate	8 fl. oz.	208
Orange drink	8 fl. oz.	110
Root beer	8 fl. oz.	104
Sprite	8 fl. oz.	95
Tab	8 fl. oz.	1
Bun:		
Regular	2.4-oz. bun	190

Food and Description	Measure or Quantity	Calories
Hot dog	1 bun	108
Junior	1.4-oz. bun	118
Steakhouse deluxe	2.4-oz. bun	190
Chicken strips:		
Adult portion	2¾ oz.	282
Child	1.4 oz.	141
Cocktail sauce	1½ oz.	57
Filet mignon	3.8 oz. (edible portion)	57
Filet of sole, fish only (See also Bun)	3-oz. piece	125
Fish, baked	4.9-oz. serving	268
Gelatin dessert	½ cup	97
Gravy, au jus	1 oz.	3
Ham & cheese:		
Bun (see Bun)		
Cheese, Swiss	2 slices (.8 oz.)	76
Ham	2½ oz.	184
Hot dog, child's, meat only (see also Bun)	1.6-oz. hot dog	140
Margarine:		
Pat	1 tsp.	36
On potato, as served	½ oz.	100
Mustard sauce, sweet & sour	1 oz.	50
New York strip steak	6.1 oz. (edible portion)	362
Onion, chopped	1 T.	4
Pickle, dill	3 slices (.7 oz.)	2
Potato:		
Baked	7.2-oz. potato	145
French fries	3-oz. serving	230
Prime ribs:		
Regular	4.2 oz. (edible portion)	286
King	6 oz. edible portion	409
Pudding, chocolate	4½ oz.	213
Ribeye	3.2 oz. (edible portion)	197
Ribeye & shrimp:		
Ribeye	3.2 oz.	197
Shrimp	2.2 oz.	139
Roll, kaiser	2.2-oz. roll	184
Salad bar:		
Bean sprouts	1 oz.	13
Broccoli	1 oz.	9
Cabbage, red	1 oz.	9
Carrots	1 oz.	12
Cauliflower	1 oz.	8
Celery	1 oz.	4
Chickpeas (Garbanzos)	1 oz.	102

Food and Description	Measure or Quantity	Calories
Mushrooms	1 oz.	8
Pepper, green	1 oz.	6
Radish	1 oz.	5
Tomato	1 oz.	6
Salad dressing:		
Blue cheese	1 oz.	129
Italian, creamy	1 oz.	138
Low calorie	1 oz.	14
Oil & vinegar	1 oz.	124
Thousand Island	1 oz.	117
Shrimp dinner	7 pieces (3½ oz.)	220
Sirloin:		
Regular	3.3 oz. (edible portion)	220
Super	6½ oz. (edible portion)	383
Tips	4 oz. (edible portion)	192
Steak sauce	1 oz.	23
Tartar sauce	1.5 oz.	285
T-Bone	4.3 oz. (edible portion)	240
Tomato (See also Salad bar):		
Slices	2 slices (.9 oz.)	5
Whole, small	3.5 oz.	22
Topping, whipped	¼ oz.	19
Worcestershire sauce	1 tsp.	4
POPCORN:		
*Plain, popped fresh:		
(Jiffy Pop)	½ of 5-oz. pkg.	244
(Jolly Time) white	1 cup	19
(Pillsbury) Microwave Popcorn:		
Regular	1 cup	70
Butter flavor	1 cup	65
Packaged:		
Buttered (Wise)	½ oz.	70
Caramel-coated:		
(Bachman)	1-oz. serving	130
(Old London) without peanuts	1¾-oz. serving	195
Cheese flavored (Bachman)	1-oz. serving	180
Cracker Jack	1-oz. serving	120
*POPOVER MIX (Flako)	1 popover	170
POPPY SEED (French's)	1 tsp.	13
POPSICLE, twin pop	3 fl. oz.	70
POP TARTS (See TOASTER CAKE OR PASTRY)		
PORK:		
Fresh:		
Chop:		
Broiled, lean & fat	3-oz. chop (weighed without bone)	332

Food and Description	Measure or Quantity	Calories
Broiled, lean only	3-oz. chop (weighed without bone)	230
Loin:		
Roasted, lean & fat	3 oz.	308
Roasted, lean only	3 oz.	216
Spareribs, braised	3 oz.	246
Cured ham:		
Roasted, lean & fat	3 oz.	246
Roasted, lean only	3 oz.	159
PORK DINNER, frozen (Swanson)	11¼-oz. dinner	290
PORK, PACKAGED (Eckrich)	1-oz. serving	45
PORK RINDS (Tom's)	.6 oz. serving	60
PORK STEAK, BREADED, frozen (Hormel)	3-oz. serving	223
PORK, SWEET & SOUR, frozen (La Choy)	½ of 15-oz. pkg.	229
PORT WINE:		
(Gallo)	3 fl. oz.	94
(Louis M. Martini)	3 fl. oz.	82
POSTUM, instant	6 fl. oz.	11
POTATO:		
Cooked:		
Au gratin	½ cup	127
Baked, peeled	2½"-dia. potato	92
Boiled, peeled	4.2-oz. potato	79
French-fried	10 pieces	156
Hash-browned, home recipe	½ cup	223
Mashed, milk & butter added	½ cup	92
Canned, solids & liq.:		
(Allen's) *Butterfield*	½ cup	45
(Del Monte)	½ cup (4 oz.)	45
Frozen:		
(Birds Eye):		
Cottage fries	2.8-oz. serving	119
Crinkle cuts, regular	3-oz. serving	115
Farm style wedge	3-oz. serving	109
French fries, regular	3-oz. serving	113
Hash browns, shredded	¼ of 12-oz. pkg.	61
Steak fries	3-oz. serving	109
Tasti Puffs	¼ of 10-oz. pkg.	192
Tiny Taters	⅕ of 16-oz. pkg.	204
Whole, peeled	3.2 oz.	59
(Green Giant):		
Sliced, in butter sauce	½ cup	80
& sweet peas in bacon cream sauce	½ cup	110
(Stouffer's):		
Au gratin	⅓ pkg.	135
Scalloped	⅓ pkg.	125
POTATO & BACON, canned (Hormel) *Short Orders,* au gratin	7½-oz. can	240

Food and Description	Measure or Quantity	Calories
POTATO & BEEF, canned,		
Dinty Moore (Hormel) *Short Orders*	1½-oz. can	250
POTATO & HAM, canned (Hormel)		
Short Orders, scalloped	7½-oz. can	250
POTATO CHIP:		
(Bachman) regular	1 oz.	160
(Featherweight) unsalted	1 oz.	160
(Frito-Lay's) natural	1 oz.	157
(Laura Scudder's)	1 oz.	150
Lay's, sour cream & onion flavor	1 oz.	160
Pringle's:		
Regular or *Cheez-Ums*	1 oz.	167
Light	1 oz.	148
(Snyder's)	1 oz.	150
(Tom's) any type	1 oz.	160
(Wise):		
Barbecue or garlic & onion	1 oz.	150
Lightly salted, natural or		
salt & vinegar	1 oz.	160
*POTATO MIX:		
Au gratin:		
(Betty Crocker)	½ cup	150
(French's) *Big Tate*, tangy	½ cup	150
(Libby's) *Potato Classics*	¾ cup	130
Creamed (Betty Crocker)	½ cup	160
Hash browns (Betty Crocker)		
with onion	½ cup	150
Hickory smoke cheese		
(Betty Crocker)	½ cup	150
Julienne (Betty Crocker) with mild		
cheese sauce	½ cup	130
Mashed:		
(American Beauty)	½ cup	120
(Betty Crocker) *Buds*	½ cup	130
(French's) *Big Tate*	½ cup	140
Scalloped:		
(Betty Crocker)	½ cup	140
(Libby's) *Potato Classics*	¾ cup	130
Sour cream & chive (Betty Crocker)	½ cup	150
*POTATO PANCAKE MIX		
(French's) *Big Tate*	3″ pancake	43
POTATO SALAD:		
Home recipe	½ cup	181
Canned (Nalley's) German style	4-oz. serving	143
POTATO STARCH		
(Manischewitz) pure	½ cup	315
POTATO STICKS (Durkee) *O & C*	1½-oz. can	231
POTATO, STUFFED, BAKED,		
frozen (Green Giant):		
With cheese flavored topping	½ of 10-oz. pkg.	200
With sour cream & chives	½ of 10-oz. pkg.	230

Food and Description	Measure or Quantity	Calories
POTATO TOPPERS (Libby's)	1 T.	30
POUND CAKE (See CAKE, Pound)		
PRESERVE OR JAM (See individual flavors)		
PRETZEL:		
(Bachman) regular or butter	1 oz.	110
(Estee) unsalted	1 piece	5
(Nabisco) *Mister Salty:*		
Dutch	1 piece	55
Mini	1 piece	7
Nuggets	1 piece	5
Twists	1 piece	22
(Rokeach)	1 oz.	110
(Snyder's) hard	1 oz.	102
(Tom's) twists	1 oz.	100
(Wise) nugget	1 oz.	110
PRODUCT 19, cereal (Kellogg's)	1 cup	110
PROSCIUTTO (Hormel) boneless	1 oz.	90
PRUNE:		
Canned:		
(Featherweight) stewed, water pack	½ cup	130
(Sunsweet) stewed	½ cup	120
Dried:		
(Del Monte) Moist Pak	2 oz.	120
(Sunsweet) whole	2 oz.	130
PRUNE JUICE:		
(Del Monte)	6 fl. oz.	120
(Mott's) regular	6 fl. oz.	140
(Sunsweet) regular	6 fl. oz.	140
PRUNE NECTAR, canned (Mott's)	6 fl. oz.	100
PUDDING OR PIE FILLING:		
Canned, regular pack:		
Banana:		
(Del Monte) *Pudding Cup*	5-oz. container	181
(Hunt's) *Snack Pack*	5-oz. container	180
(Thank You Brand)	½ cup	150
Butterscotch:		
(Del Monte) *Pudding Cup*	5-oz. container	184
(Thank You Brand)	½ cup	149
Chocolate:		
(Del Monte) *Pudding Cup*	5-oz. container	201
(Hunt's) *Snack Pack*	5-oz. container	180
(Thank You Brand)	½ cup	191
Rice (Comstock; Menner's)	½ of 7½-oz. can	120
Tapioca:		
(Del Monte) *Pudding Cup*	5-oz. container	172
(Hunt's) *Snack Pack*	5-oz. container	140
Vanilla (Del Monte)	5-oz. container	188
Canned, dietetic pack:		
(Estee)	½ cup	70

Food and Description	Measure or Quantity	Calories
(Sego)	4-oz. serving	125
Chilled, *Swiss Miss:*		
Butterscotch, chocolate malt or vanilla	4-oz. container	150
Chocolate or double rich	4-oz. container	160
Tapioca	4-oz. container	130
Frozen (Rich's):		
Banana	3-oz. container	142
Butterscotch or vanilla	4½-oz. container	199
Chocolate	4½-oz. container	214
*Mix, sweetened, regular & instant:		
Banana:		
(Jello-O) cream, regular	½ cup	161
(Royal) regular	½ cup	160
Butter pecan (Jello-O) instant	½ cup	175
Butterscotch:		
(Jell-O) instant	½ cup	175
(My-T-Fine) regular	½ cup	143
Chocolate:		
(Jell-O) regular	½ cup	174
(My-T-Fine) regular	½ cup	169
Coconut:		
(Jell-O) cream, regular	½ cup	176
(Royal) instant	½ cup	170
Flan (Royal) regular	½ cup	150
Lemon:		
(Jell-O) instant	½ cup	170
(My-T-Fine) regular	½ cup	164
Lime (Royal) Key Lime, regular	½ cup	160
Pineapple (Jell-O) cream, instant	½ cup	176
Pistachio (Jell-O) instant	½ cup	174
Raspberry (Salada) *Danish Dessert*	½ cup	176
Rice, *Jell-O Americana*	½ cup	176
Strawberry (Salada) *Danish Dessert*	½ cup	130
Tapioca:		
Jell-O Americana, chocolate	½ cup	173
(My-T-Fine) vanilla	½ cup	130
Vanilla:		
(Jell-O) French, regular	½ cup	172
(Royal)	½ cup	180
*Mix, dietetic:		
Butterscotch:		
(D-Zerta)	½ cup	68
(Featherweight) artificially sweetened	½ cup	60
(Royal) instant	½ cup	100
Chocolate:		
(Dia-Mel)	½ cup	50

Food and Description	Measure or Quantity	Calories
(Estee)	½ cup	70
(Royal) instant	½ cup	100
Lemon:		
(Dia-Mel)	½ cup	53
(Estee)	½ cup	106
Vanilla:		
(Dia-Mel)	½ cup	50
(D-Zerta)	½ cup	71
(Featherweight) artifically sweetened	½ cup	60
PUDDING STIX (Good Humor)	1¾-fl.-oz. pop	90
PUFFED RICE:		
(Malt-O-Meal)	1 cup	50
(Quaker)	1 cup	55
PUFFED WHEAT:		
(Malt-O-Meal)	1 cup	50
(Quaker)	1 cup	54
PUMPKIN, canned (Libby's) solid pack	½ cup	80
PUMPKIN SEED, in hull	1 oz.	116

Q

QUAIL, raw, meat & skin	4 oz.	195
QUIK, (Nestlé) chocolate or strawberry	1 tsp.	45
QUISP, cereal	1⅙ cup	121

R

RADISH	2 small radishes	4
RAISIN, dried:		
(Del Monte) golden	3 oz.	260
(Sun-Maid)	1 oz.	290
RAISINS, RICE & RYE, cereal (Kellogg's)	¾ cup	140
RALSTON, cereal	¼ cup	90
RASPBERRY:		
Fresh:		
Black, trimmed	½ cup	49
Red, trimmed	½ cup	41
Frozen (Birds Eye) quick thaw	5-oz. serving	155
RASPBERRY PRESERVE OR JAM:		
Sweetened (Smucker's)	1 T.	53

Food and Description	Measure or Quantity	Calories
Dietetic:		
(Estee, Louis Sherry)	1 T.	6
(Featherweight) red	1 T.	16
(S&W) *Nutradiet,* red	1 T.	12
RATATOUILLE, frozen (Stouffer's)	5-oz. serving	60
RAVIOLI:		
Canned, regular pack (Franco-American) beef, *RavioliOs*	7½-oz. serving	210
Canned, dietetic (Estee) beef	8-oz. can	210
Frozen:		
(Celentano):		
Regular	ʊ½ oz.	410
Mini	4 oz.	250
(Weight Watchers) baked	8¹⁄₁₆ oz. meal	290
RELISH:		
Dill (Vlasic)	1 oz.	2
Hamburger:		
(Heinz)	1 oz.	30
(Vlasic)	1 T.	24
Hot dog:		
(Heinz)	1 oz.	35
(Vlasic)	1 T.	28
Sweet (Vlasic)	1 T.	18
RENNET MIX (Junket):		
*Powder, any flavor:		
Made with skim milk	½ cup	90
Made with whole milk	½ cup	120
Tablet	1 tablet	1
RHINE WINE:		
(Great Western)	3 fl. oz.	73
(Taylor)	3 fl. oz.	75
RHUBARB, cooked, sweetened	½ cup	169
***RICE:**		
Brown (Uncle Ben's) parboiled, with added butter	⅔ cup	152
White:		
(Minute Rice) instant, no added butter	⅔ cup	120
(Success) long grain	½ cooking bag	110
White & wild (Carolina)	½ cup	90
RICE, FRIED (See also RICE MIX):		
*Canned (La Choy)	⅓ of 11-oz. can	190
Frozen:		
(Birds Eye)	3.7-oz. serving	104
(Green Giant) *Boil 'N Bag*	10-oz. entree	300
(La Choy) & pork	8-oz. serving	280
RICE, FRIED, SEASONING MIX (Kikkoman)	1-oz. pkg.	91
***RICE KRINKLES,** cereal (Post)	⅞ cup	109

Food and Description	*Measure or Quantity*	*Calories*
RICE KRISPIES, cereal (Kellogg's):		
Regular, frosted, cocoa or strawberry	1 oz.	110
Marshmallow	1 oz.	140
RICE MIX:		
Beef:		
*(Carolina) *Bake-It-Easy*	¼ pkg.	110
*(Lipton) & sauce	½ cup	160
*(Minute Rice)	½ cup	149
Rice-A-Roni	⅙ pkg.	130
Chicken:		
*(Carolina) *Bake-It-Easy*	¼ pkg.	110
*(Lipton) & sauce	½ cup	150
Rice-A-Roni	⅙ pkg.	130
*Fried (Minute Rice)	½ cup	156
*Herb & butter (Lipton)	½ cup	160
*Long grain & wild (Minute Rice)	½ cup	148
*Mushroom (Lipton) & sauce	½ cup	140
*Oriental (Carolina) *Bake-It-Easy*	½ of pkg.	120
Spanish:		
*(Carolina) *Bake-It-Easy*	¼ of pkg.	110
*(Minute Rice)	½ cup	150
Rice-A-Roni	⅐ pkg.	110
***RICE SEASONING** (French's)		
Spice Your Rice:		
Beef flavor & onion or cheese & chives	½ cup	160
Buttery herb	½ cup	170
RICE, SPANISH:		
canned:		
Regular pack (Comstock; Menner's)	½ of 7½-oz. can	140
Dietetic (Featherweight) low sodium	7½-oz. serving	140
Frozen (Birds Eye)	3.7-oz. serving	122
RICE & VEGETABLE, frozen:		
(Birds Eye):		
French style	3.7-oz. serving	117
Peas with mushrooms	2⅓ oz.	109
(Green Giant) *Rice Originals*		
& broccoli in cheese sauce	½ cup	140
Pilaf	½ cup	120
RICE WINE:		
Chinese, 20.7% alcohol	1 fl. oz.	38
Japanese, 10.6% alcohol	1 fl. oz.	72
ROCK & RYE (Mr. Boston)	1 fl. oz.	75
ROE, baked or broiled, cod & shad	4 oz.	143
ROLL OR BUN:		
Commercial type, non-frozen:		
Biscuit (Wonder)	1¼-oz. piece	80
Brown & serve (Wonder)		
Gem Style	1-oz. piece	80

Food and Description	Measure or Quantity	Calories
Club (Pepperidge Farm)	1.3-oz. piece	100
Crescent (Pepperidge Farm) butter	1-oz. piece	110
Croissant (Pepperidge Farm):		
Butter, cinnamon or honey-sesame	2-oz. piece	200
Chocolate	2.4-oz. piece	260
Walnut	2-oz. piece	210
Dinner:		
Home Pride	1-oz. piece	85
(Pepperidge Farm)	.7-oz. piece	60
Finger (Pepperidge Farm) sesame or poppy seed	.6-oz. piece	60
Frankfurter:		
(Arnold) Hot Dog	1.3-oz. piece	100
(Pepperidge Farm)	1¾-oz. piece	110
(Wonder)	1-oz. piece	80
French:		
(Arnold) *Francisco*, sourdough	1.1-oz. piece	90
(Pepperidge Farm):		
Small	1.3-oz. piece	110
Large	3-oz. piece	240
Golden Twist (Pepperidge Farm)	1-oz. piece	110
Hamburger:		
(Arnold)	1.4-oz. piece	110
(Pepperidge Farm)	1.5-oz. piece	130
Roman Meal	1.8-oz. piece	193
Hoagie (Wonder)	5-oz. piece	400
Old fashioned (Pepperidge Farm)	.6-oz. piece	60
Parkerhouse (Pepperidge Farm)	.6-oz. piece	50
Party (Pepperidge Farm)	.4-oz. piece	30
Sandwich (Arnold) soft	1.3-oz. piece	110
Soft (Pepperidge Farm)	1¼-oz. piece	110
Frozen:		
Apple crunch (Sara Lee)	1-oz. piece	102
Caramel pecan (Sara Lee)	1.3-oz. piece	161
Cinnamon (Sara Lee)	.9-oz. piece	100
Croissant (Sara Lee)	.9-oz. piece	109
Crumb (Sara Lee) French	1¾-oz. piece	188
Danish (Sara Lee):		
Apple	1.3-oz. piece	120
Cheese	1.3-oz. piece	130
Cinnamon raisin	1.3-oz. piece	147
Pecan	1.3-oz. piece	148
Honey (Morton) mini	1.3-oz. piece	133
*ROLL OR BUN DOUGH:		
Frozen (Rich's):		
Cinnamon	2¼-oz. piece	173
Frankfurter	1 piece	136
Hamburger, regular	1 piece	134
Parkerhouse	1 piece	82

Food and Description	Measure or Quantity	Calories
Refrigerated (Pillsbury):		
Apple danish, *Pipin' Hot*	1 piece	250
Caramel danish, with nuts	1 piece	155
Cinnamon raisin danish	1 piece	145
Crescent	1 piece	100
White, bakery style	1 piece	100
*ROLL MIX, HOT (Pillsbury)	1 piece	100
ROMAN MEAL CEREAL	⅓ cup	103
ROSEMARY LEAVES (French's)	1 tsp.	5
ROSÉ WINE:		
Corbett Canyon (Glenmore)	3 fl. oz.	63
(Great Western)	3 fl. oz.	80
(Paul Masson):		
Regular, 11.8% alcohol	3 fl. oz.	76
Light, 7.1% alcohol	3 fl. oz.	49
ROY ROGERS:		
Bar Burger, R.R.	1 burger	611
Biscuit	1 biscuit	231
Breakfast crescent sandwich:		
Regular	4.5-oz. sandwich	401
With bacon	4.7-oz. sandwich	431
With ham	5.8-oz. sandwich	557
With sausage	5.7-oz. sandwich	449
Brownie	1 piece	264
Cheeseburger:		
Regular	1 burger	563
With bacon	1 burger	581
Chicken:		
Breast	1 piece	412
Leg	1 piece	140
Thigh	1 piece	296
Wing	1 piece	192
Coleslaw	3½-oz. serving	110
Danish:		
Apple	1 piece	249
Cheese	1 piece	254
Cherry	1 piece	271
Drinks:		
Coffee, black	6 fl. oz.	Tr.
Coke:		
Regular	12 fl. oz.	145
Diet	12 fl. oz.	1
Hot chocolate	6 fl. oz.	123
Milk	8 fl. oz.	150
Orange juice:		
Regular	7 fl. oz.	99
Large	10 fl. oz.	136
Shake:		
Chocolate	1 shake	358
Strawberry	1 shake	306
Vanilla	1 shake	315

Food and Description	Measure or Quantity	Calories
Tea, iced, plain	8 fl. oz.	0
Egg & biscuit platter:		
Regular	1 meal	394
With bacon	1 meal	435
With ham	1 meal	442
With sausage	1 meal	550
Hamburger	1 burger	456
Pancake platter, with syrup & butter		
Plain	1 order	452
With bacon	1 order	493
With ham	1 order	506
With sausage	1 order	608
Potato:		
Baked, *Hot Topped:*		
Plain	1 potato	211
With bacon & cheese	1 potato	397
With broccoli & cheese	1 potato	376
With margarine	1 potato	274
With sour cream & chives	1 potato	408
With taco beef & cheese	1 potato	463
French fries:		
Regular	3 oz.	268
Large	4 oz.	357
Potato salad	3½-oz. order	107
Roast beef sandwich:		
Plain:		
Regular	1 sandwich	317
Large	1 sandwich	360
With cheese:		
Regular	1 sandwich	424
Large	1 sandwich	467
Salad bar:		
Bacon bits	1 T.	33
Beets, sliced	¼ cup	16
Broccoli	½ cup	20
Carrot, shredded	¼ cup	42
Cheese, cheddar	¼ cup	112
Croutons	1 T.	35
Egg, chopped	1 T.	27
Lettuce	1 cup	10
Macaroni salad	1 T.	30
Mushrooms	¼ cup	5
Noodle, Chinese	¼ cup	55
Pepper, green	1 T.	2
Potato salad	1 T.	25
Tomato	1 slice	7
Salad dressing:		
Regular:		
Bacon & tomato	1 T.	68
Bleu cheese	1 T.	75
Ranch	1 T.	77

Food and Description	Measure or Quantity	Calories
1,000 Island	1 T.	80
Low calorie, Italian	1 T.	35
Strawberry shortcake	7.2-oz. serving	447
Sundae:		
Caramel	1 sundae	293
Hot fudge	1 sundae	337
Strawberry	1 sundae	216
RUTABAGA:		
Canned (Sunshine) solids & liq.	½ cup	32
Frozen (Sunshine)	4 oz.	50

S

Food and Description	Measure or Quantity	Calories
SAFFLOWER SEED, in hull	1 oz.	89
SAGE (French's)	1 tsp.	4
SAKE WINE	1 fl. oz.	39
SALAD CRUNCHIES (Libby's)	1 T.	35
SALAD DRESSING:		
Regular:		
Bacon (Seven Seas) creamy	1 T.	60
Bacon & tomato (Henri's)	1 T.	70
Bleu or blue cheese		
(Wish-Bone) chunk	1 T.	70
Caesar:		
(Pfeiffer)	1 T.	70
(Seven Seas) *Viva*	1 T.	60
Capri (Seven Seas)	1 T.	70
Cheddar & bacon (Wish-Bone)	1 T.	70
Cucumber (Wish-Bone)	1 T.	80
French:		
(Bernstein's) creamy	1 T.	56
(Henri's):		
Hearty	1 T.	70
Original	1 T.	60
(Seven Seas) creamy	1 T.	60
(Wish-Bone) garlic or herbal	1 T.	60
Garlic (Wish-Bone) creamy	1 T.	80
Green Goddess (Seven Seas)	1 T.	60
Herb & spice (Seven Seas)	1 T.	60
Italian:		
(Bernstein's)	1 T.	50
(Henri's):		
Authentic	1 T.	80
Creamy garlic	1 T.	50
(Pfeiffer) chef	1 T.	60
(Seven Seas) *Viva!*	1 T.	70
(Wish-Bone) regular, or herbal	1 T.	70

Food and Description	Measure or Quantity	Calories
Miracle Whip (Kraft)	1 T.	70
Ranchouse (Henri's) *Chef's Recipe*	1 T.	70
Red wine vinegar & oil (Seven Seas)	1 T.	60
Roquefort:		
(Bernstein's)	1 T.	65
(Marie's)	1 T.	105
Russian:		
(Henri's)	1 T.	60
(Pfeiffer)	1 T.	65
(Wish-Bone)	1 T.	45
Sour cream & bacon (Wish-Bone)	1 T.	70
Spin Blend (Hellmann's)	1 T.	57
Thousand Island:		
(Pfeiffer)	1 T.	65
(Wish-Bone) plain	1 T.	70
Vinaigrette (Bernstein's) French	1 T.	49
Dietetic or low calorie:		
Bacon & tomato (Estee)	1 T.	8
Bleu or blue cheese:		
(Estee)	1 T.	8
(Featherweight) imitation	1 T.	4
(Herni's)	1 T.	30
(Tillie Lewis) *Tasti-Diet*	1 T.	12
(Walden Farms) chunky	1 T.	27
(Wish-Bone) chunky	1 T.	40
Buttermilk (Wish-Bone)	1 T.	50
Caesar:		
(Estee) garlic	1 T.	4
(Featherweight) creamy	1 T.	14
Catalina (Kraft)	1 T.	16
Chef's Recipe Ranchouse (Henri's)	1 T.	30
Cucumber (Kraft)	1 T.	30
French:		
(Estee)	1 T.	4
(Featherweight) low calorie	1 T.	6
(Henri's) original	1 T.	40
(Walden Farms)	1 T.	33
(Wish-Bone)	1 T.	30
Herb & spice (Featherweight)	1 T.	6
Garlic (Estee)	1 T.	2
Italian:		
(Estee) creamy	1 T.	6
(Henri's) creamy	1 T.	25
(Kraft) zesty	1 T.	6
(Walden Farms)	1 T.	9
(Weight Watchers)	1 T.	50
(Wish-Bone)	1 T.	30
Onion & chive (Wish-Bone)	1 T.	40
Onion & cucumber (Estee)	1 T.	6
Red wine/vinegar (Featherweight)	1 T.	6

Food and Description	Measure or Quantity	Calories
Russian:		
(Featherweight) creamy	1 T.	6
(Weight Watchers)	1 T.	50
(Wish-Bone)	1 T.	25
Tas-Tee (Henri's)	1 T.	30
Thousand Island:		
(Estee)	1 T.	6
(Henri's)	1 T.	30
(Kraft)	1 T.	30
(Walden Farms)	1 T.	24
(Weight Watchers)	1 T.	50
(Wish-Bone)	1 T.	40
2-Calorie Low Sodium		
(Featherweight)	1 T.	2
Whipped (Tillie Lewis) *Tasti Diet*	1 T.	18
Yoganaise (Henri's)	1 T.	60
SALAD DRESSING MIX:		
*Regular (Good Seasons):		
Blue cheese	1 T.	84
Buttermilk, farm style	1 T.	58
Farm style	1 T.	53
French, old fashioned	1 T.	83
Garlic, cheese	1 T.	85
Garlic & herb	1 T.	84
Italian, regular, cheese or zesty	1 T.	84
Dietetic:		
*Blue cheese (Weight Watchers)	1 T.	10
*French (Weight Watchers)	1 T.	4
Garlic (Dia-Mel)	½-oz. pkg.	21
*Italian:		
(Good Seasons) regular	1 T.	8
(Weight Watchers):		
Regular	1 T.	2
Creamy	1 T.	4
*Russian (Weight Watchers)	1 T.	4
*Thousand Island		
(Weight Watchers)	1 T.	12
SALAD SUPREME (McCormick)	1 tsp.	11
SALAMI:		
(Eckrich) for beer or cooked	1 oz.	70
(Hormel):		
Beef	1 slice	40
Genoa, DiLusso	1-oz. serving	100
Hard, sliced	1 slice	34
(Oscar Mayer):		
For beer, beef	.8-oz. slice	66
Cotto	.8-oz. slice	54
Genoa	.3-oz. slice	35
SALISBURY STEAK, frozen:		
(Armour) *Classic Lite*	10-oz. meal	290
(Banquet):		
Buffet Supper	2-lb. pkg.	1260

Food and Description	Measure or Quantity	Calories
Man Pleaser	19-oz. dinner	1024
(Stouffer's) *Lean Cuisine*	9½-oz. pkg.	270
(Swanson):		
Regular:		
Dinner, 4-compartment	11-oz. dinner	460
Entree	5½-oz. entree	370
Hungry Man	16½-oz. dinner	710
Main Course	8½-oz. entree	430
(Weight Watchers) beef, Romano	8¾-oz. meal	300
SALMON:		
Baked or broiled	6¾″ × 2½″ × 1″ piece	264
Canned, regular pack, solids & liq.:		
Keta (Bumble Bee)	½ cup	153
Pink or Humpback:		
(Bumble Bee)	½ cup	155
(Del Monte)	7¾-oz. can	290
Sockeye or Red or Blueback:		
(Bumble Bee)	½ cup	188
(Libby's)	7¾-oz. can	380
Canned, dietetic (S&W) *Nutradiet,* low sodium	½ cup	188
SALMON, SMOKED (Vita):		
Lox, drained	4-oz. jar	136
Nova, drained	4-oz. can	221
SALT:		
(Morton):		
Regular	1 tsp.	0
Lite	1 tsp.	0
Substitute:		
(Adolph's) plain	1 tsp.	1
(Morton) plain	1 tsp.	Tr.
Salt-It (Estee)	1 tsp.	0
SALT 'N SPICE SEASONING (McCormick)	1 tsp.	3
SANDWICH SPREAD:		
(Hellmann's)	1 T.	65
(Oscar Mayer)	1-oz. serving	67
SANGRIA (Taylor)	3 fl. oz.	99
SARDINE, canned:		
Atlantic (Del Monte) with tomato sauce	7½-oz. can	319
Imported (Underwood) in mustard or tomato sauce	3¾-oz. can	220
Norwegian:		
(Granadaisa Brand) in tomato sauce	3¾-oz. can	195
(King David Brand) brisling in olive oil	3¾-oz. can	293
(Queen Helga Brand) in sild oil	3¾-oz. can	310
SAUCE:		
Regular:		
A-1	1 T.	12

Food and Description	Measure or Quantity	Calories
Barbecue:		
Chris & Pitt's	1 T.	15
(Gold's)	1 T.	25
(Heinz)	¼ cup	80
(Kraft) plain or hot	¼ cup	80
Open Pit (General Foods) original, hot n' spicy or smoke flavor	1 T.	24
Burrito (Del Monte)	¼ cup	20
Chili (See CHILI SAUCE)		
Cocktail:		
(Gold's)	1 T.	31
(Pfeiffer)	1-oz. serving	100
Escoffier Sauce Diable	1 T.	20
Escoffier Sauce Robert	1 T.	20
Famous Sauce	1 T.	69
Hot, *Frank's*	1 tsp.	1
Italian (See also SPAGHETTI SAUCE or TOMATO SAUCE):		
(Contadina)	4-oz. serving	71
(Ragú) red cooking	3½-oz. serving	45
Salsa Mexicana (Contadina)	4 fl. oz.	38
Salsa Picante (Del Monte) regular	¼ cup	20
Salsa Roja (Del Monte)	¼ cup	20
Seafood cocktail (Del Monte)	1 T.	21
Soy:		
(Chun King)	1 T.	5
(Gold's)	1 T.	10
(Kikkoman) light	1 T.	9
(La Choy)	1 T.	8
Spare rib (Gold's)	1 T.	51
Steak (Dawn Fresh) with mushrooms	1-oz. serving	9
Steak Supreme	1 T.	20
Sweet & sour:		
(Chun King)	1.8 oz.	57
(Contadina)	4 fl. oz.	150
(La Choy)	1-oz. serving	51
Swiss steak (Carnation)	2-oz. serving	20
Tabasco	¼ tsp.	Tr.
Taco:		
Old El Paso, hot or mild	1 T.	5
(Ortega) hot or mild	1 oz.	13
Tartar:		
(Hellmann's)	1 T.	73
(Nalley's)	1 T.	89
Teriyaki (Kikkoman)	1 T.	12
V-8	1-oz. serving	25
White, medium	¼ cup	103
Worcestershire:		
(French's) regular or smoky	1 T.	10

Food and Description	Measure or Quantity	Calories
(Gold's)	1 T.	42
Dietetic (Estee):		
Barbecue	1 T.	16
Cocktail	1 T.	10
Taco	1 oz.	14
SAUCE MIX:		
Regular:		
A la King (Durkee)	1-oz. pkg.	133
*Cheese:		
(Durkee)	½ cup	168
(French's)	½ cup	160
Hollandaise:		
(Durkee)	1-oz. pkg.	173
*(French's)	1 T.	15
*Sour cream (French's)	2½ T.	60
*Sweet & sour (Kikkoman)	1 T.	18
Teriyaki (Kikkoman)	1.5-oz. pkg.	125
*White (Durkee)	1 cup	238
*Dietetic (Weight Watchers) lemon butter	1 T.	8
SAUERKRAUT, canned:		
(Claussen) drained	½ cup	16
(Comstock) regular	½ cup	30
(Del Monte) solids & liq.	1 cup	55
(Silver Floss) solids & liq.:		
Regular	½ cup	30
Krispy Kraut	½ cup	25
(Vlasic)	2 oz.	8
SAUSAGE:		
*Brown & Serve (Hormel)	1 sausage	70
Patty (Hormel)	1 patty	150
Polish-style:		
(Eckrich)	1-oz. serving	95
(Hormel) *Kilbase*	1-oz. serving	122
Pork:		
(Eckrich)	1-oz. link	100
*(Hormel) *Little Sizzlers*	1 link	51
(Jimmy Dean)	2-oz. serving	227
*(Oscar Mayer) *Little Friers*	1 link	82
Roll (Eckrich) minced	1-oz. slice	80
Smoked:		
(Eckrich) beef, *Smok-Y-Links*	.8-oz. link	70
(Hormel) smokies	1 sausage	80
(Oscar Mayer) beef	1½-oz. link	123
*Turkey (Louis Rich) links or tube	1-oz. serving	45
Vienna:		
(Hormel) regular	1 sausage	50
(Libby's) in barbecue sauce	2½-oz. serving	180
SAUTERNE:		
(Great Western)	3 fl. oz.	79
(Taylor)	3 fl. oz.	81

Food and Description	Measure or Quantity	Calories
SCALLOP:		
Steamed	4-oz. serving	127
Frozen:		
(Mrs. Paul's) breaded & fried	3½-oz. serving	210
(Stouffer's) *Lean Cuisine*	11-oz. pkg.	230
SCHNAPPS, APPLE (Mr. Boston)	1 fl. oz.	78
SCHNAPPS, PEPPERMINT		
(Mr. Boston)	1 fl. oz.	115
SCREWDRIVER COCKTAIL		
(Mr. Boston) 12½% alcohol	3 fl. oz.	111
SCROD DINNER OR ENTREE,		
frozen (Gorton's) *Light Recipe*	1 pkg.	260
SEAFOOD NEWBERG, frozen:		
(Armour) *Dinner Classics*	10½-oz. meal	280
(Mrs. Paul's)	8½ oz.	310
SEAFOOD PLATTER, frozen		
(Mrs. Paul's) breaded & fried	9-oz. serving	510
SEGO DIET FOOD, canned:		
Regular	10-fl.-oz. can	225
Lite	10-fl.-oz. can	150
SELTZER (Canada Dry)	Any quantity	0
SERUTAN	1 tsp.	6
SESAME SEEDS (French's)	1 tsp.	9
7-GRAIN CEREAL		
(Loma Linda)	1 oz.	110
SHAD, CREOLE	4-oz. serving	172
SHAKE 'N BAKE:		
Chicken, original	1 pkg.	282
Crispy country mild	1 pkg.	309
Fish	2-oz. pkg.	232
Italian	1 pkg.	289
Pork, barbecue	1 pkg.	306
SHAKEY'S		
Chicken, fried, & potatoes:		
3-piece	1 order	947
5-piece	1 order	1700
Ham & cheese sandwich	1 sandwich	550
Pizza:		
Cheese:		
Thin	13" pizza	1403
Thick	13" pizza	1890
Onion, green pepper, olive & mushroom:		
Thin	13" pizza	1713
Thick	13" pizza	2200
Pepperoni:		
Thin	13" pizza	1833
Thick	13" pizza	2320
Sausage & mushroom:		
Thin	13" pizza	1759
Thick	13" pizza	2256

Food and Description	Measure or Quantity	Calories
Sausage & pepperoni:		
Thin	13" pizza	2111
Thick	13" pizza	2598
Special:		
Thin	13" pizza	2110
Thick	13" pizza	2597
Potatoes	15-piece order	950
Spaghetti with meat sauce & garlic bread	1 order	940
Super hot hero	1 sandwich	810
SHELLS, PASTA, STUFFED, frozen:		
(Celentano):		
Broccoli & cheese	11½-oz. pkg.	400
Cheese:		
Without sauce	½ of 12½-oz. pkg.	350
With sauce	½ of 16-oz. pkg.	320
(Stouffer's) cheese stuffed	9-oz. serving	320
***SHELLS AND SAUCE** (Lipton):*		
Creamy garlic	½ cup	200
Herb tomato	½ cup	170
SHERBET OR SORBET:		
Cassis (Häagen-Dazs)	4 fl. oz.	128
Daiquiri Ice (Häagen-Dazs)	4 fl. oz.	136
Lemon (Häagen-Dazs)	4 fl. oz.	140
Orange:		
(Baskin-Robbins)	4 fl. oz.	158
(Häagen-Dazs)	4 fl. oz.	140
SHERRY:		
Cocktail (Gold Seal)	3 fl. oz.	122
Cream (Great Western) Solera	3 fl. oz.	141
Dry (Williams & Humbert)	3 fl. oz.	120
Dry Sack (Williams & Humbert)	3 fl. oz.	120
SHREDDED WHEAT:		
(Nabisco):		
Regular size	¾-oz. biscuit	90
Spoon Size	⅔ cup	110
(Quaker)	1 biscuit	52
(Sunshine):		
Regular	1 biscuit	90
Bite size	⅔ cup	110
SHRIMP:		
Canned (Bumble Bee) solids & liq.	4½-oz. can	90
Frozen (Mrs. Paul's):		
Breaded & fried	3 oz.	190
Parmesan	11-oz. meal	310
SHRIMP COCKTAIL canned or frozen (Sau-Sea)	4 oz.	113
SHRIMP DINNER, frozen:		
(Armour) *Classic Lites,* in sherried cream sauce	10½-oz. meal	280
(Blue Star) *Dining Lite,* creole	10-oz. meal	210

119

Food and Description	Measure or Quantity	Calories
(Conagra) *Light & Elegant*	10-oz. meal	218
(Stouffer's) Newberg	6½-oz. serving	300
SLENDER (Carnation):		
Bar	1 bar	135
Dry	1 packet	110
Liquid	10-fl.-oz. can	220
SLOPPY HOT DOG SEASONING MIX (French's)	1½-oz. pkg.	160
SLOPPY JOE:		
Canned:		
(Hormel) *Short Orders*	7½-oz. can	340
(Libby's):		
Beef	⅓ cup	110
Pork	⅓ cup	120
Frozen (Banquet) *Cookin' Bag*	5-oz. pkg.	199
SLOPPY JOE SAUCE (Ragú) *Joe Sauce*	3½ oz.	50
SLOPPY JOE SEASONING MIX:		
*(Durkee) pizza flavor	1¼ cups	746
(French's)	1 pkg.	128
SMURF BERRY CRUNCH, cereal (Post)	1 cup	116
SNACK BAR (Pepperidge Farm):		
Apple nut, apricot-raspberry or blueberry	1.7-oz. piece	170
Brownie nut or date nut	1½-oz. piece	190
Chocolate chip or coconut macaroon	1½-oz. piece	210
SNO BALL (Hostess)	1 piece	149
SOAVE WINE (Antinori)	3 fl. oz.	84
SOFT DRINK:		
Sweetened:		
Apple (Slice)	6 fl. oz.	98
Birch beer (Canada Dry)	6 fl. oz.	82
Bitter lemon:		
(Canada Dry)	6 fl. oz.	75
(Schweppes)	6 fl. oz.	82
Bubble Up	6 fl. oz.	73
Cactus Cooler (Canada Dry)	6 fl. oz.	90
Cherry:		
(Canada Dry) wild	6 fl. oz.	98
(Shasta) black	6 fl. oz.	81
Cherry-lime (Spree)	6 fl. oz.	79
Chocolate (Yoo-Hoo)	6 fl. oz.	93
Club	Any quantity	0
Cola:		
Coca-Cola:		
Regular or caffeine-free	6 fl. oz.	71
Classic	6 fl. oz.	61
Jamaica (Canada Dry)	6 fl. oz.	79
Pepsi-Cola, regular or *Pepsi Free*	6 fl. oz.	80
(Shasta) regular	6 fl. oz.	72

Food and Description	Measure or Quantity	Calories
(Slice)	6 fl. oz.	82
(Spree)	6 fl. oz.	73
Collins mix (Canada Dry)	6 fl. oz.	60
Cream:		
(Canada Dry) vanilla	6 fl. oz.	97
(Schweppes)	6 fl. oz.	86
Dr. Nehi (Royal Crown)	6 fl. oz.	82
Dr. Pepper	6 fl. oz.	75
Fruit punch:		
(Nehi)	6 fl. oz.	99
(Shasta)	6 fl. oz.	87
Ginger ale:		
(Canada Dry) regular	6 fl. oz.	68
(Fanta)	6 fl. oz.	60
(Shasta)	6 fl. oz.	60
(Spree)	6 fl. oz.	60
Ginger beer (Schweppes)	6 fl. oz.	70
Grape:		
(Fanta)	6 fl. oz.	81
(Hi-C)	6 fl. oz.	74
(Nehi)	6 fl. oz.	96
(Schweppes)	6 fl. oz.	95
(Welch's) sparkling	6 fl. oz.	90
Grapefruit (Spree)	6 fl. oz.	77
Half & half (Canada Dry)	6 fl. oz.	82
Hi-Spot (Canada Dry)	6 fl. oz.	75
Lemon lime:		
(Minute Maid)	6 fl.oz.	67
(Shasta)	6 fl. oz.	73
(Spree)	6 fl. oz.	77
Lemon-tangerine (Spree)	6 fl. oz.	82
Mello Yello	6 fl. oz.	81
Mountain Dew	6 fl. oz.	89
Mr. PiBB	6 fl. oz.	68
Orange:		
(Canada Dry) *Sunrise*	6 fl. oz.	97
(Hi-C)	6 fl. oz.	74
(Slice)	6 fl. oz.	97
(Sunkist)	6 fl. oz.	96
Peach (Nehi)	6 fl. oz.	101
Pineapple (Canada Dry)	6 fl. oz.	82
Quinine or tonic water		
(Canada Dry; Schweppes)	6 fl. oz.	68
Root beer:		
Barrelhead (Canada Dry)	6 fl. oz.	82
(Dad's)	6 fl. oz.	83
Rooti (Canada Dry)	6 fl. oz.	79
(Shasta) draft	6 fl. oz.	77
(Spree)	6 fl. oz.	77
7-Up	6 fl. oz.	72
Slice	6 fl. oz.	76
Sprite	6 fl. oz.	68

Food and Description	Measure or Quantity	Calories
Strawberry (Shasta)	6 fl. oz.	73
Tahitian Treat (Canada Dry)	6 fl. oz.	97
Tropical blend (Spree)	6 fl. oz.	73
Upper Ten (Royal Crown)	6 fl. oz.	84
Dietetic:		
Apple (Slice)	6 fl. oz.	2
Birch beer (Shasta)	6 fl. oz.	2
Bubble Up	6 fl. oz.	1
Cherry (Shasta) black	6 fl. oz.	<0
Chocolate (Shasta)	6 fl. oz.	0
Coffee (No-Cal)	6 fl. oz.	1
Cola:		
(Canada Dry; Shasta)	6 fl. oz.	0
Coca-Cola, regular or caffeine free	6 fl. oz.	<1
Diet Rite	6 fl. oz.	<1
Pepsi, diet, light or caffeine free	6 fl. oz.	<1
(Slice)	6 fl. oz.	10
Cream (Shasta)	6 fl. oz.	<1
Dr. Pepper	6 fl. oz.	<2
Fresca	6 fl. oz.	2
Ginger Ale:		
(Canada Dry)	6 fl. oz.	1
(No-Cal)	6 fl. oz.	0
Grape (Shasta)	6 fl. oz.	0
Grapefruit (Shasta)	6 fl. oz.	2
Lemon-lime (Minute Maid)	6 fl.oz.	9
Mr. PiBB	6 fl. oz.	<1
Orange:		
(Canada Dry; No-Cal)	6 fl. oz.	1
(Minute Maid)	6 fl. oz.	8
(Shasta)	6 fl. oz.	<1
Quinine or tonic (No-Cal)	6 fl. oz.	3
RC 100 (Royal Crown) caffeine free	6 fl. oz.	<1
Red Pop (Shasta)	*6 fl. oz.*	*0*
Root beer:		
Barrelhead (Canada Dry)	6 fl. oz.	1
(Dad's; Ramblin'; Shasta)	6 fl. oz.	<1
7-Up	6 fl. oz.	2
Slice	6 fl. oz.	13
Sprite	6 fl. oz.	1
Tab, regular or caffeine free	6 fl. oz.	<1
SOLE, frozen:		
(Mrs. Paul's) fillets, breaded & fried	6-oz. serving	280
(Van De Kamp's) batter dipped, french fried	1 piece	140
(Weight Watchers) in lemon sauce	9⅛-oz. meal	200

Food and Description	Measure or Quantity	Calories
SOUFFLE, frozen (Stouffer's):		
Cheese	6-oz. serving	355
Corn	4-oz. serving	155
SOUP:		
Canned, regular pack:		
*Asparagus (Campbell), condensed, cream of:		
Regular	8-oz. serving	90
Creamy Natural	8-oz. serving	200
Bean:		
(Campbell):		
Chunky, with ham, old fashioned	11-oz. can	290
*Condensed, with bacon	8-oz. serving	150
(Grandma Brown's)	8-oz. serving	182
Bean, black:		
*(Campbell) condensed	8-oz. serving	110
(Crosse & Blackwell)	6½-oz. serving	80
Beef:		
(Campbell):		
Chunky:		
Regular	10¾-oz. can	190
Stroganoff	10¾-oz. can	300
*Condensed:		
Regular	8-oz. serving	80
Broth	8-oz. serving	15
Consommé	8-oz. serving	25
Noodle, home style	8-oz. serving	90
(College Inn) broth	1 cup	18
(Swanson) Broth	7¼-oz. can	20
*Broccoli (Campbell) condensed, *Creamy Natural*	8-oz. serving	140
Celery:		
*(Campbell) condensed, cream of	8-oz. serving	100
*(Rokeach):		
Prepared with milk	10-oz. serving	190
Prepared with water	10-oz. serving	90
*Cheddar cheese (Campbell)	8-oz. serving	130
Chicken:		
(Campbell):		
Chunky:		
& rice	19-oz. can	280
vegetable	19-oz. can	340
*Condensed:		
Alphabet	8-oz. serving	80
Broth:		
Plain	8-oz. serving	35
& rice	8-oz. serving	50
Cream of	8-oz. serving	110
Gumbo	8-oz. serving	60

Food and Description	Measure or Quantity	Calories
Mushroom, creamy	8-oz. serving	120
Noodle:		
Regular	8-oz. serving	70
NoodleOs	8-oz. serving	70
& rice	8-oz. serving	60
Vegetable	8-oz. serving	70
*Semi-condensed, *Soup For One*,		
Vegetable, full flavored	11-oz. serving	120
(College Inn) broth	1 cup	35
(Swanson) broth	7¼-oz. can	30
Chili beef (Campbell) *Chunky*	11-oz. can	290
Chowder:		
Beef'n vegetable (Hormel) *Short Orders*	7½-oz. can	120
Clam:		
Manhattan style:		
(Campbell):		
Chunky	19-oz. can	300
*Condensed	8-oz. serving	70
(Crosse & Blackwell)	6½-oz. serving	50
New England style:		
*(Campbell):		
Condensed:		
Made with milk	8-oz. serving	150
Made with water	8-oz. serving	80
Semi-condensed, *Soup for One:*		
Made with milk	11-oz. serving	190
Made with water	11-oz. serving	130
(Crosse & Blackwell)	6½-oz. serving	90
*(Gorton's)	1 can	560
Ham'n potato (Hormel)	7½-oz. can	130
Consommé madrilene (Crosse & Blackwell)	6½-oz. serving	25
Crab (Crosse & Blackwell)	6½-oz. serving	50
Gazpacho (Crosse & Blackwell)	6½-oz. serving	30
Ham'n butter bean (Campbell) *Chunky*	10¾-oz. can	280
Lentil (Crosse & Blackwell) with ham	6½-oz. serving	80
*Meatball alphabet (Campbell) condensed	8-oz. serving	100
Minestrone:		
(Campbell):		
Chunky	19-oz. can	280
*Condensed	8-oz. serving	80
(Crosse & Blackwell)	6½-oz. serving	90
Mushroom:		
*(Campbell):		
Condensed:		
Cream of	8-oz. serving	100

124

Food and Description	Measure or Quantity	Calories
Golden	8-oz. serving	80
(Crosse & Blackwell) cream of, bisque	6½-oz. serving	90
*(Rokeach) cream of:		
Prepared with milk	10-oz. serving	240
Prepared with water	10-oz. serving	150
*Noodle (Campbell) & ground beef	8-oz. serving	90
*Onion (Campbell):		
Regular	8-oz. serving	60
Cream of:		
Made with water	8-oz. serving	100
Made with water & milk	8-oz. serving	140
*Oyster stew (Campbell):		
Made with milk	8-oz. serving	150
Made with water	8-oz. serving	80
*Pea, green (Campbell)	8-oz. serving	160
Pea, split:		
(Campbell):		
Chunky, with ham	19-oz. can	400
*Condensed, with ham & bacon	8-oz. serving	160
(Grandma Brown's)	8-oz. serving	184
*Pepper pot (Campbell)	8-oz. serving	90
*Potato (Campbell) cream of:		
Regular:		
Made with water	8-oz. serving	70
Made with water & milk	8-oz. serving	110
Creamy Natural	8-oz. serving	220
Shav (Gold's)	8-oz. serving	11
Shrimp:		
*(Campbell) condensed, cream of:		
Made with milk	8-oz. serving	160
Made with water	8-oz. serving	90
(Crosse & Blackwell)	6½-oz. serving	90
*Spinach (Campbell) condensed, *Creamy Natural*	8-oz. serving	160
Steak & potato (Campbell) *Chunky*	19-oz. can	340
Tomato:		
(Campbell):		
Condensed:		
Regular:		
Made with milk	8-oz. serving	160
Made with water	8-oz. serving	90
& rice, old fashioned	8-oz. serving	110
Creamy Natural	8-oz. serving	190
Semi-condensed, *Soup For One,* Royale	11-oz. serving	180
*(Rokeach):		
Made with milk	10-oz. serving	190

Food and Description	Measure or Quantity	Calories
Made with water	10-oz. serving	90
Turkey (Campbell) *Chunky*	18¾-oz. can	300
Vegetable:		
(Campbell):		
Chunky:		
Regular	19-oz. can	260
Beef, old fashioned	19-oz. can	320
*Condensed:		
Regular	8-oz. serving	80
Beef or vegetarian	10-oz. serving	70
*Semi-condensed,		
Soup For One, old world	11-oz. serving	160
*(Rokeach) vegetarian	10-oz. serving	90
Vichyssoise (Crosse & Blackwell)	6½-oz. serving	70
*Won ton (Campbell)	8-oz. serving	40
Canned, dietetic pack:		
Beef (Campbell) *Chunky,*		
& mushroom, low sodium	10¾-oz. can	210
Chicken:		
(Campbell) low sodium:		
Regular, with noodles	10¾-oz. can	160
Vegetable	10¾-oz. can	240
*(Estee) & vegetable	7½-oz. serving	120
*Minestrone (Estee)	7½-oz. serving	160
Mushroom (Campbell) cream of,		
low sodium	10½-oz. can	200
Onion (Campbell) low sodium	10½-oz. can	80
Pea, split (Campbell) low sodium	10¾-oz. can	240
Tomato: (Campbell) low sodium		
with tomato pieces	10½-oz. can	180
Vegetable (Campbell) *Chunky*		
low sodium	10¾-oz. can	170
Frozen:		
*Barley & mushroom		
(Mother's Own)	8-oz. serving	50
Chowder, clam, New England style		
(Stouffer's)	8-oz. serving	200
Pea, split:		
*(Mother's Own)	8-oz. serving	130
(Stouffer's)	8¼-oz. serving	190
Spinach (Stouffer's) cream of	8-oz. serving	230
*Won ton (La Choy)	½ of 15-oz. pkg.	50
Mix, regular:		
Beef:		
Carmel Kosher	6 fl. oz.	12
*(Lipton) *Cup-A-Soup:*		
Noodle	6 fl. oz.	45
Lots-A-Noodles	7 fl. oz.	120
*(Weight Watchers) broth	6 fl. oz.	10
*Chicken:		
Carmel Kosher	6 fl. oz.	12

Food and Description	Measure or Quantity	Calories
(Lipton):		
Cup-A-Broth	6 fl. oz.	25
Cup-A-Soup, & rice	6 fl. oz.	45
Country style, hearty	6 fl. oz.	70
Lots-A-Noodles, regular	7 fl. oz.	120
*Minestrone (Manischewitz)	6 fl. oz.	50
*Mushroom:		
Carmel Kosher	6 fl. oz.	12
(Lipton):		
Regular, beef	8 fl. oz.	40
Cup-A-Soup, cream of	6 fl. oz.	80
*Noodle (Lipton):		
With chicken broth	8 fl. oz.	70
Giggle Noodle	8 fl. oz.	80
*Onion:		
Carmel Kosher	6 fl. oz.	12
(Lipton):		
Regular, beef	8 fl. oz.	35
Cup-A-Soup	6 fl. oz.	30
*Pea, green (Lipton) *Cup-A-Soup*	6 fl. oz.	120
*Pea, split (Manischewitz)	6 fl. oz.	45
*Tomato (Lipton) *Cup-A-Soup*	6 fl. oz.	80
*Tomato onion (Lipton)	8 fl. oz.	80
*Vegetable:		
(Lipton):		
Regular, country	8 fl. oz.	80
Cup-A-Soup:		
Regular, spring	6 fl. oz.	40
Country style, harvest	6 fl. oz.	90
Lots-A-Noodles, garden	7 fl. oz.	130
(Manischewitz)	6 fl. oz.	50
(Southland) frozen	⅕ of 16-oz. pkg.	60
*Mix, dietetic:		
(Estee):		
Beef noodle	6 fl. oz.	20
Chicken noodle	6 fl. oz.	25
Tomato	6 fl. oz.	40
(Lipton) *Cup-A-Soup-Trim*	6 fl. oz.	10
SOUP GREENS (Durkee)	2⅓-oz. jar	216
SOUTHERN COMFORT:		
80 proof	1 fl. oz.	79
100 proof	1 fl. oz.	95
SOYBEAN CURD OR TOFU	2¾″ × 1½″ × 1″ cake	86
SOYBEAN OR NUT:		
Dry roasted (*Soy Ahoy: Soy Town*)	1 oz.	139
Oil roasted (*Soy Ahoy; Soy Town*)		
plain, barbecue or garlic	1 oz.	152
SPAGHETTI:		
Cooked:		
8-10 minutes, "Al Dente"	1 cup	216
14-20 minutes, tender	1 cup	155

127

Food and Description	Measure or Quantity	Calories
Canned:		
(Franco-American):		
In meat sauce	7½-oz. can	210
With meatballs in tomato sauce, *SpaghettiOs*	7⅜-oz. can	210
With sliced franks in tomato sauce, *SpaghettiOs*	7⅜-oz. can	210
(Hormel) *Short Orders*, & meatballs in tomato sauce	7½-oz. can	210
(Libby's) & meatballs in tomato sauce	7½-oz. serving	189
Dietetic (Estee) & meatballs	7½-oz. serving	240
Frozen:		
(Armour) *Dinner Classics*, with meatballs	11-oz. meal	350
(Banquet) & meat sauce	8-oz. pkg.	270
(Conagra) *Light & Elegant*, & meat sauce	10¼-oz. entree	290
(Morton) & meatball	11-oz. dinner	360
(Stouffer's) *Lean Cuisine*	11½-oz. pkg.	280
(Weight Watchers) with meat sauce	10½-oz. meal	280
SPAGHETTI SAUCE, canned:		
Regular pack:		
Garden Style (Ragú)	4-oz. serving	80
Marinara:		
(Prince)	4-oz. serving	80
(Ragú)	5-oz. serving	120
Meat or meat flavored:		
(Prego)	4-oz. serving	150
(Prince)	½ cup	101
(Ragú) regular	4-oz. serving	80
Meatless or plain:		
(Prego)	4-oz. serving	140
(Ragú) regular	4-oz. serving	80
Mushroom:		
(Hain)	4-oz. serving	80
(Prego Plus)	4-oz. serving	130
(Ragú) Extra Thick & Zesty	4-oz. serving	110
Sausage & green pepper (Prego Plus)	4-oz. serving	170
Veal (Prego Plus)	4-oz. serving	150
Dietetic pack:		
(Furman's) low sodium	½ cup	83
(Prego) low sodium	½ cup	100
***SPAGHETTI SAUCE MIX:**		
(Durkee) regular	½ cup	45
(French's) with mushrooms	⅝ cup	100
(Spatini)	½ cup	84
SPAM, luncheon meat (Hormel):		
Regular, smoke flavored or with		

Food and Description	Measure or Quantity	Calories
cheese chunks	1-oz. serving	85
Deviled	1 T.	35
SPARKLING COOLER CITRUS,		
La Croix (Heileman)	6 fl. oz.	107
SPECIAL K, cereal (Kellogg's)	1 cup	110
SPINACH:		
Fresh, whole leaves	½ cup	4
Boiled	½ cup	18
Canned, regular pack (Allens)		
solids & liq.	½ cup	25
Canned, dietetic pack (Del Monte)		
No Salt Added	½ cup	25
Frozen:		
(Birds Eye):		
Chopped or leaf	⅓ pkg.	28
Creamed	⅓ pkg.	60
(Green Giant):		
Creamed	½ cup	70
Harvest Fresh	4-oz. serving	30
(McKenzie) chopped or cut	⅓ pkg.	25
(Stouffer's) souffle	4-oz. serving	135
SPINACH PUREE, canned		
(Larsen) low sodium	½ cup	22
SQUASH, SUMMER:		
Yellow, boiled slices	½ cup	13
Zucchini, boiled slices	½ cup	9
Canned (Del Monte) zucchini, in		
tomato sauce	½ cup	30
Frozen:		
(Birds Eye) zucchini	⅓ pkg.	19
(McKenzie) crookneck	⅓ pkg.	20
(Mrs. Paul's) sticks,		
batter dipped, french fried	⅓ pkg.	180
SQUASH, WINTER:		
Acorn, baked	½ cup	56
Hubbard, baked, mashed	½ cup	51
Frozen:		
(Birds Eye)	⅓ pkg.	43
(Southland) butternut	4-oz. serving	45
STEAK (See BEEF)		
STEAK & GREEN PEPPERS, frozen:		
(Green Giant)	9-oz. entree	250
(Swanson)	8½-oz. entree	200
STEAK UMM	2 oz.	180
STOCK BASE (French's) beef		
or chicken	1 tsp.	8
STRAWBERRY:		
Fresh, capped	½ cup	26
Frozen (Birds Eye):		
Halves	⅓ pkg.	164
Whole	¼ pkg.	89

Food and Description	Measure or Quantity	Calories
Whole, quick thaw	½ pkg.	125
STRAWBERRY DRINK (Hi-C):		
Canned	6 fl. oz.	89
*Mix	6 fl. oz.	68
STRAWBERRY FRUIT JUICE, canned (Smucker's)	8 fl. oz.	120
STRAWBERRY KRISPIES, cereal (Kellogg's)	¾ cup	110
STRAWBERRY NECTAR, canned (Libby's)	6 fl. oz.	60
STRAWBERRY PRESERVE OR JAM:		
Sweetened:		
(Smucker's)	1 T.	53
(Welch's)	1 T.	52
Dietetic or low calorie:		
(Estee; Louis Sherry)	1 T.	6
(Diet Delight)	1 T.	12
(Featherweight) calorie reduced	1 T.	16
STUFFING MIX:		
*Beef, *Stove Top*	½ cup	181
*Chicken:		
(Bell's)	½ cup	190
Stove Top	½ cup	178
*Cornbread, *Stove Top*	½ cup	174
Cube or herb seasoned (Pepperidge Farm)	1 oz.	110
*Pork, *Stove Top*	½ cup	176
*Premium Blend (Bell's)	½ cup	180
*Ready Mix (Bell's)	½ cup	224
White bread (Mrs. Cubbison's)	1 oz.	101
STURGEON, smoked	4-oz. serving	169
SUCCOTASH:		
Canned:		
(Comstock) whole kernel	½ cup	80
(Libby's) cream style	½ cup	111
(Stokely-Van Camp)	½ cup	85
Frozen:		
(Birds Eye)	⅓ pkg.	104
(Frosty Acres)	3.3 oz.	100
SUGAR:		
Brown	1 T.	48
Confectioners'	1 T.	30
Granulated	1 T.	46
Maple	1¾" × 1¼" × ½" piece	104
SUGAR CORN POPS, cereal (Kellogg's)	1 cup	110
SUGAR CRISP, cereal (Post)	⅞ cup	112
SUGAR PUFFS, cereal (Malt-O-Meal)	⅞ cup	110
SUGAR SMACKS, cereal (Kellogg's)	¾ cup	110

Food and Description	Measure or Quantity	Calories
SUGAR SUBSTITUTE:		
(Estee)	1 tsp.	12
(Featherweight)	3 drops	0
Sprinkle Sweet (Pillsbury)	1 tsp.	2
Sweet'n-it (Estee) liquid	5 drops	0
*SUKIYAKI DINNER (Chun King)		
stir fry	6 oz.	257
SUNFLOWER SEED (Fisher):		
In hull, roasted, salted	1 oz.	86
Hulled, dry roasted, salted	1 oz.	164
Hulled, oil roasted, salted	1 oz.	167
SUZY Q (Hostess):		
Banana	1 piece	240
Chocolate	1 piece	240
SWEETBREADS, calf, braised	4-oz. serving	191
SWEET POTATO:		
Baked, peeled	5" × 1" potato	155
Canned, (Allen's)	4-oz. serving	50
Frozen:		
(Mrs. Paul's) candied, with apples	4-oz. serving	150
(Stouffer's) & apples	5-oz. serving	160
SWISS STEAK, frozen (Swanson)	10-oz. dinner	350
SWORDFISH, broiled	3" × 3" × ½" steak	218
SYRUP (See also TOPPING):		
Regular:		
Apricot (Smucker's)	1 T.	50
Blackberry (Smucker's)	1 T.	50
Chocolate or chocolate-flavored:		
Bosco	1 T.	55
(Hershey's)	1 T.	40
(Nestlé) *Quik*	1 oz.	80
Corn, *Karo,* dark or light	1 T.	58
Maple, *Karo,* imitation	1 T.	57
Pancake or waffle:		
(Aunt Jemima)	1 T.	53
Golden Griddle	1 T.	54
Karo	1 T.	58
Log Cabin, regular or buttered	1 T.	56
Mrs. Butterworth's	1 T.	55
Strawberry (Smucker's)	1 T.	50
Dietetic or low calorie:		
Blueberry (Estee)	1 T.	4
Chocolate or chocolate-flavored		
(Diet Delight)	1 T.	8
Coffee (No-Cal)	1 T.	6
Cola (No-Cal)	1 T.	0
Maple (S&W) *Nutradiet*	1 T.	12
Pancake or waffle:		
(Aunt Jemima)	1 T.	29
(Cary's)	1 T.	6
(Estee)	1 T.	4
(Featherweight)	1 T.	12

T

Food and Description	Measure or Quantity	Calories
TACO:		
*(Ortega)	1 oz.	54
*Mix (Durkee)	½ cup	321
Shell (Ortega)	1 shell	50
TACO BELL RESTAURANTS:		
Bellbeefer:		
Regular	5-oz. serving	280
With cheese and tomato	5½-oz. serving	305
Burrito:		
Bean	7.2-oz. serving	440
Beef	6.7-oz. serving	430
Combination	8.4-oz. serving	350
Crispas, cinnamon	2.2-oz. serving	230
Enchirato	6.5-oz. serving	325
Nachos:		
Regular	3.3-oz. serving	355
Bellgrande	10.6-oz. serving	725
Pintos and cheese	5.1-oz. serving	225
Taco:		
Regular	3.1-oz. serving	210
Light	5-oz. serving	345
Taco salad	1 serving	910
Tostada, beef	7.4-oz. serving	360
TAMALE:		
Canned:		
(Hormel) beef, *Short Orders*	7½-oz. can	270
Old El Paso, with chili gravy	1 tamale	96
Frozen (Hormel) beef	1 tamale	130
TANG, orange, regular	6 fl. oz.	87
TANGERINE OR MANDARIN ORANGE:		
Fresh (Sunkist)	1 large tangerine	39
Canned, solids & liq.:		
Regular pack (Dole)	½ cup	76
Dietetic pack:		
(Diet Delight) juice pack	½ cup	50
(Featherweight) water pack	½ cup	35
(S&W) *Nutradiet*	½ cup	28
TANGERINE DRINK, canned (Hi-C)	6 fl. oz.	90
TANGERINE JUICE, frozen (Minute Maid)	6 fl. oz.	85
TAPIOCA, dry, *Minute,* quick-cooking	1 T.	32
TAQUITO, frozen (Van de Kamp's) beef	8-oz. serving	490

Food and Description	Measure or Quantity	Calories
TARRAGON (French's)	1 tsp.	5
TASTEEOS, cereal (Ralston Purina)	1¼ cups	110
*TEA:		
Bag:		
(Lipton):		
Plain or flavored	1 cup	2
Herbal:		
Almond pleasure or cinnamon apple	1 cup	2
Quietly chamomile or toasty spice	1 cup	6
(Sahadi) spearmint	1 cup	4
Instant (Nestea)100%	6 fl. oz.	0
TEAM, cereal	1 cup	110
TEA MIX, ICED:		
*(Lipton) lemon & sugar flavored	1 cup	60
***Nestea,** lemon-flavored	1 cup	6
*Dietetic, **Crystal Light**	8 fl. oz.	2
TEQUILA SUNRISE COCKTAIL, (Mr. Boston) 12½% alcohol	3 fl. oz.	120
TERIYAKI, frozen (Stouffer's)	10-oz. serving	365
TERIYAKI BASTE & GLAZE (Kikkoman)	1 T.	28
*TEXTURED VEGETABLE PROTEIN,		
Morningstar Farms:		
Breakfast link	1 link	73
Breakfast patties	1 patty	100
Breakfast strips	1 strip	37
Grillers	1 patty	190
THURINGER:		
(Eckrich) **Smoky Tang**	1-oz. serving	80
(Hormel):		
Beefy	1-oz. serving	100
Old Smokehouse	1-oz. serving	100
(Louis Rich) turkey	1-oz. serving	50
(Oscar Mayer)	.8-oz. slice	73
TIGER TAILS (Hostess)	2¼-oz. piece	210
TOASTED WHEAT AND RAISINS, cereal (Nabisco)	1 oz.	100
TOASTER CAKE OR PASTRY:		
Pop-Tarts (Kellogg's):		
Regular:		
Blueberry, brown sugar cinnamon or cherry	1 pastry	210
Strawberry	1 pastry	200
Frosted:		
Blueberry, chocolate fudge or strawberry	1 pastry	200
Brown sugar cinnamon, cherry,	1 pastry	210
Chocolate-vanilla creme	1 pastry	220

Food and Description	Measure or Quantity	Calories
Toaster Strudel (Pillsbury)	1 slice	190
Toastettes (Nabisco) regular or frosted	1 piece	200
Toast-R-Cake (Thomas'):		
Blueberry	1 piece	108
Bran	1 piece	103
Corn	1 piece	120
TOASTIES, cereal (Post)	1¼ cups	107
TOASTY O'S, cereal (Malt-O-Meal)	1¼ cup	110
TOFUTTI:		
Frozen:		
Regular:		
Chocolate supreme or wildberry supreme	4 fl. oz.	210
Maple walnut	4 fl. oz.	230
Vanilla	4 fl. oz.	200
Cuties:		
Chocolate	1 piece	140
Vanilla	1 piece	130
Lite Lite	4 fl. oz.	90
Love Drops:		
Cappuccino or chocolate	4 fl. oz.	230
Vanilla	4 fl. oz.	220
Soft serve:		
Regular	4 fl. oz.	158
Hi-Lite:		
Chocolate	4 fl. oz.	100
Vanilla	4 fl. oz.	90
TOMATO:		
Regular, whole	1 med. tomato	33
Cherry, whole	4 pieces	14
Canned, regular pack, solids & liq.:		
(Contadina) sliced, baby	½ cup	50
(Del Monte) stewed	4 oz.	37
(Stokely-Van Camp) stewed	½ cup	35
Canned, dietetic pack, solids & liq.:		
(Del Monte) No Salt Added	½ cup	35
(Featherweight)	½ cup	20
(Furman's) low sodium	½ cup	72
TOMATO & PEPPER, HOT CHILI, *Old El Paso,* Jalapeño	¼ cup	13
TOMATO JUICE, CANNED:		
Regular pack:		
(Campbell; Libby's)	6-fl.-oz. can	35
(Del Monte)	6-fl.-oz. can	36
(Musselman's)	6-fl.-oz. can	30
(Welch's)	6 fl. oz.	35
Dietetic pack (Diet Delight; Featherweight)	6 fl. oz.	35

Food and Description	Measure or Quantity	Calories
TOMATO JUICE COCKTAIL, canned:		
(Ocean Spray) *Firehouse Jubilee*	6 fl. oz.	44
SnapE-Tom	6 fl. oz.	40
TOMATO PASTE, canned:		
Regular pack:		
(Contadina) Italian	6-oz. serving	210
(Del Monte)	6-oz. can	150
Dietetic (Featherweight) low sodium	6-oz. can	150
TOMATO, PICKLED (Claussen) green	1 piece	6
TOMATO PUREE, canned:		
Regular (Contadina) heavy	1 cup	100
Dietetic (Featherweight)	1 cup	90
TOMATO SAUCE, canned:		
(Contadina) regular	1 cup	90
(Del Monte):		
Regular or No Salt Added	1 cup	70
Hot	½ cup	40
With tomato bits	1 cup	92
(Furman's)	½ cup	58
(Hunt's) with cheese	4-oz. serving	70
TOM COLLINS (Mr. Boston) 12½% alcohol	3 fl. oz.	111
***TOM COLLINS MIX,** (Bar-Tender's)	6 fl. oz.	177
TONGUE, beef, braised	4-oz. serving	277
TOPPING:		
Regular:		
Butterscotch (Smucker's)	1 T.	70
Caramel (Smucker's)regular	1 T.	70
Chocolate fudge (Hershey's)	1 T.	50
Nut (Planters)	1 oz.	180
Pecans in syrup (Smucker's)	1 T.	65
Pineapple (Smucker's)	1 T.	65
Strawberry (Smucker's)	1 T.	60
Walnuts in syrup (Smucker's)	1 T.	65
Dietetic, chocolate (Diet Delight)	1 T.	16
TOPPING, WHIPPED:		
Regular:		
Cool Whip (Birds Eye) dairy	1 T.	16
Lucky Whip, aerosol	1 T.	12
Whip Topping (Rich's)	¼ oz.	20
Dietetic (Featherweight)	1 T.	3
*Mix:		
Regular, *Dream Whip*	1 T.	5
Dietetic (D-Zerta; Estee)	1 T.	4
***TOP RAMEN,** beef (Nissin Foods)	3-oz. serving	390
TORTILLA (Amigos)	6″ × ⅛″ tortilla	111
TOSTADA, frozen (Van de Kamp's)	8½-oz. serving	530
TOSTADA SHELL (*Old El Paso*)	1 shell	57

Food and Description	Measure or Quantity	Calories
TOTAL, cereal	1 cup	110
TRIPE, canned (Libby's)	6-oz. serving	290
TRIPLE SEC LIQUEUR		
(Mr. Boston)	1 fl. oz.	79
TRIX, cereal (General Mills)	1 cup	110
TUNA:		
Canned in oil:		
(Bumble Bee):		
Chunk, light, solids & liq.	½ cup	265
Solid, white, solids & liq.	½ cup	285
(Carnation) solids & liq.	6½-oz. can	427
Canned in water:		
(Breast O'Chicken)	6½-oz. can	211
(Bumble Bee):		
Chunk, light, solids & liq.	½ cup	117
Solid, white, solids & liq.	½ cup	126
(Featherweight) light, chunk	6½-oz. can	210
*****TUNA HELPER** (General Mills):		
Country dumplings or noodles cheese	⅓ pkg.	230
Creamy noodle	⅓ pkg.	280
TUNA PIE, frozen:		
(Banquet)	8-oz. pie	395
(Morton)	8-oz. pie	370
TUNA SALAD:		
Home recipe	4-oz. serving	193
Canned (Carnation)	¼ of 7½-oz. can	100
TURF & SURF DINNER, frozen		
(Armour) *Classic Lights*	10-oz. meal	250
TURKEY:		
Barbecued (Louis Rich) breast, half	1 oz.	40
Packaged:		
(Carl Buddig):		
Regular	1 oz.	50
Ham or salami	1 oz.	40
(Hormel) breast	1 slice	30
(Louis Rich):		
Turkey bologna	1-oz. slice	60
Turkey cotto salami	1-oz. slice	50
Turkey ham, chopped	1-oz. slice	45
Turkey pastrami	1-oz. slice	35
(Oscar Mayer) breast	7½-oz. slice	21
Roasted:		
Flesh & skin	4-oz. serving	253
Dark meat	2½" × 1⅝" × ¼" slice	43
Light meat	4" × 2" × ¼" slice	75
Smoked (Louis Rich):		
Drumsticks	1 oz. (without bone)	40
Wing drumettes	1 oz. (without bone)	45
TURKEY DINNER OR ENTREE,		
frozen:		
(Banquet):		
American Favorites	11-oz. dinner	320

Food and Description	Measure or Quantity	Calories
Extra Helping	9-oz. dinner	723
(Conagra) *Light & Elegant,* sliced	8-oz. entree	230
(Le Menu) sliced breast, with mushrooms	11¼-oz. dinner	460
(Morton)	11¼-oz. dinner	279
(Swanson):		
Regular	8¾-oz. entree	250
Hungry Man	18½-oz. dinner	590
(Weight Watchers) stuffed, breast	8½-oz. meal	260
TURKEY PIE, frozen:		
(Banquet):		
Regular	8-oz. pie	526
Supreme	8-oz. pie	430
(Morton)	8-oz. pie	340
(Stouffer's)	10-oz. pie	460
(Swanson) chunk	10-oz. pie	530
TURKEY TETRAZZINI, frozen:		
(Stouffer's)	6-oz. serving	240
(Weight Watchers)	10-oz. pkg.	310
TURNIP GREENS, canned (Allen's) chopped, solids & liq.	½ cup	20
TURNIP ROOTS, frozen (McKenzie) diced	1 oz.	4
TURNOVER:		
Frozen (Pepperidge Farm):		
Apple or cherry	1 turnover	310
Blueberry, peach or raspberry	1 turnover	320
Refrigerated (Pillsbury)	1 turnover	170
TWINKIE (Hostess)	1 piece	160

U

UFO'S, canned (Franco-American):		
Regular	7½ oz.	180
With meteors	7½ oz.	240

V

VALPOLICELLA WINE (Antinori)	3 fl. oz.	84
VANDERMINT, liqueur	1 fl. oz.	90
VANILLA EXTRACT (Virginia Dare)	1 tsp.	10

Food and Description	Measure or Quantity	Calories
VEAL, broiled, medium cooked:		
Loin chop	4 oz.	265
Rib, roasted	4 oz.	305
Steak or cutlet, lean & fat	4 oz.	245
VEAL DINNER, frozen:		
(Armour) *Dinner Classics,*		
parmigiana	10¾-oz. meal	400
(Morton) Light	11-oz. dinner	290
(Swanson) parmigiana,		
Hungry Man	20-oz. dinner	640
(Weight Watchers) parmigiana,		
2-compartment	8.625-oz. meal	230
VEAL STEAK, frozen (Hormel):		
Regular	4-oz. serving	130
Breaded	4-oz. serving	240
VEGETABLE BOUILLON		
(Herb-Ox):		
Cube	1 cube	6
Packet	1 packet	12
VEGETABLE JUICE COCKTAIL:		
Regular, *V-8*	6 fl. oz.	35
Dietetic:		
(S&W) *Nutradiet,* low sodium	6 fl. oz.	35
V-8, low sodium	6 fl. oz.	40
VEGETABLES IN PASTRY,		
frozen (Pepperidge Farm):		
Asparagus with mornay sauce or		
broccoli with cheese	3¾ oz.	250
Cauliflower & cheese sauce	3¾ oz.	220
Spinach almondine	3¾ oz.	260
Zucchini provencal	3¾ oz.	210
VEGETABLES, MIXED:		
Canned, regular pack:		
(Del Monte) solids & liq.	½ cup	40
(La Choy):		
Chinese	⅓ of 14-oz. pkg.	12
Chop Suey	½ cup	10
(Libby's) solids & liq.	½ cup	40
Canned, dietetic pack:		
(Featherweight)	½ cup	40
(Larsen) *Fresh-Lite*	½ cup	35
Frozen:		
(Birds Eye):		
Regular:		
Broccoli, cauliflower &		
carrots in butter sauce	⅓ pkg.	51
Carrots, peas & onions,		
deluxe	⅓ pkg.	52
Medley, in butter sauce	⅓ of 10-oz. pkg.	62
Farm Fresh:		
Broccoli, cauliflower &		

Food and Description	Measure or Quantity	Calories
carrot strips	⅓ pkg.	30
Brussels sprouts, cauliflower & carrots	⅓ pkg.	38
International Style:		
Chinese style	⅓ pkg.	85
Mexican style	⅓ pkg.	133
Stir Fry, Chinese style	⅓ pkg.	36
(Chun King) chow mein, drained	4 oz.	32
(Frosty Acres):		
Regular	3.3 oz.	65
Dutch	3.2 oz.	30
Oriental	3.2 oz.	25
Soup mix	3 oz.	45
Stew	3 oz.	42
Swiss mix	3 oz.	25
(Green Giant):		
Regular:		
Broccoli, cauliflower & carrots in cheese sauce	½ cup	60
Corn, broccoli bounty	½ cup	60
Harvest Fresh	½ cup	60
Harvest Get Togethers:		
Broccoli-cauliflower medley	½ cup	60
Broccoli fanfare	½ cup	80
(Le Sueur) peas, onions & carrots in butter sauce	½ cup	90
(Southland):		
Gumbo	⅓ of 16-oz. pkg.	40
Stew	4 oz.	60
VEGETABLE STEW, canned *Dinty Moore* (Hormel)	7½-oz. serving	170
"VEGETARIAN FOODS":		
Canned or dry:		
Chicken, fried (Loma Linda) with gravy	1½-oz. piece	70
Chili (Worthington)	½ cup	177
Choplet (Worthington)	1 choplet	50
Dinner cuts (Loma Linda) drained	1 piece	60
Dinner loaf (Loma Linda)	¼ cup	50
Franks, big (Loma Linda)	1.9-oz. frank	100
Franks, sizzle (Loma Linda)	2.2-oz. frank	85
FriChik (Worthington)	1 piece	75
Little links (Loma Linda) drained	.8-oz. link	40
Non-meatballs (Worthington)	1 meatball	32
Nuteena (Loma Linda)	½" slice	160
Patty mix (Loma Linda)	¼ cup	50
Prime Stakes	1 slice	171
Proteena (Loma Linda)	½" slice	140
Sandwich spread (Loma Linda)	1 T.	23

Food and Description	Measure or Quantity	Calories
*Soyagen, all purpose powder (Loma Linda)	1 cup	130
Soyameat (Worthington):		
Beef, sliced	1 slice	44
Chicken, diced	1 oz.	40
Soyameal, any kind (Worthington)	1 oz.	120
Stew pack (Loma Linda) drained	2 oz.	70
Super links (Worthington)	1 link	110
Swiss steak with gravy (Loma Linda)	1 steak	140
Vegelona (Loma Linda)	½" slice	100
Vega-links (Worthington)	1 link	55
Wheat protein	4 oz.	124
Worthington 209	1 slice	58
Frozen:		
Beef pie (Worthington)	1 pie	278
Bologna (Loma Linda)	1 oz.	75
Chicken, fried (Loma Linda)	2-oz. serving	180
Chic-Ketts (Worthington)	1 oz.	53
Corned beef, sliced (Worthington)	1 slice	32
Fri Pats (Worthington)	1 patty	204
Meatballs (Loma Linda)	1 meatball	63
Meatless salami (Worthington)	1 slice	44
Prosage (Worthington)	1 link	60
Smoked beef, slices (Worthington)	1 slice	14
Wham, roll (Worthington)	1 slice	36
VERMOUTH:		
Dry & extra dry (Lejon; Noilly Pratt)	1 fl. oz.	33
Sweet (Lejon; Taylor)	1 fl. oz.	45
VICHY WATER (Schweppes)	Any quantity	0
VINEGAR	1 T.	2

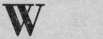

WAFFELOS, cereal (Ralston Purina)	1 cup	110
WAFFLE, frozen:		
(Aunt Jemima) jumbo	1 waffle	86
(Eggo):		
Apple cinnamon	1 waffle	150
Blueberry or strawberry	1 waffle	130
Home style	1 waffle	120
WALNUT, English or Persian (Diamond A)	1 cup	679

Food and Description	Measure or Quantity	Calories
WALNUT FLAVORING, black		
(Durkee) imitation	1 tsp.	4
WATER CHESTNUT, canned:		
(Chun King) whole, drained	½ of 8½-oz. can	85
(La Choy) drained	¼ cup	16
WATERCRESS, trimmed	½ cup	3
WATERMELON:		
Wedge	4″ × 8″ wedge	111
Diced	½ cup	21
WELSH RAREBIT:		
Home recipe	1 cup	415
Frozen:		
(Green Giant)	5-oz. serving	219
(Stouffer's)	5-oz. serving	355
WENDY'S		
Bacon, breakfast	1 strip	55
Bacon cheeseburger on white bun	1 burger	460
Breakfast sandwich	1 sandwich	370
Buns:		
Wheat, multi-grain	1 bun	135
White	1 bun	160
Chicken sandwich on multi-grain bun	1 sandwich	320
Chili:		
Regular	8 oz.	260
Large	12 oz.	390
Condiments:		
Bacon	½ strip	30
Cheese, American	1 slice	70
Onion rings	.3-oz. piece	4
Pickle, dill	4 slices	1
Relish	.3-oz. serving	14
Tomato	1 slice	2
Danish	1 piece	360
Drinks:		
Coffee	6 fl. oz.	2
Cola:		
Regular	12 fl. oz	110
Dietetic	12 fl. oz.	Tr.
Fruit flavored drink	12 fl. oz.	110
Hot chocolate	6 fl. oz.	100
Milk:		
Regular	8 fl. oz.	150
Chocolate	8 fl. oz.	210
Non-cola	12 fl. oz.	100
Orange juice	6 fl. oz.	80
Egg, scrambled	1 order	190
Frosty dairy dessert:		
Small	12 fl. oz.	400
Medium	16 fl. oz.	533
Large	20 fl. oz.	667

Food and Description	Measure or Quantity	Calories
Hamburger:		
Double, on white bun	1 burger	560
Kids Meal	1 burger	220
Single:		
On wheat bun	1 burger	340
On white bun	1 burger	350
Omelet:		
Ham & cheese	1 omelet	250
Ham, cheese & mushroom	1 omelet	290
Mushroom, onion & green pepper	1 omelet	210
Potato:		
Baked, hot stuffed:		
Plain	1 potato	250
Broccoli & cheese	1 potato	500
Cheese	1 potato	590
Chicken à la King	1 potato	350
Sour cream & chives	1 potato	460
Stroganoff & sour cream	1 potato	490
French fries	regular order	280
Home fries	1 order	360
Salad Bar, *Garden Spot*:		
Alfalfa sprouts	2 oz.	20
Bacon bits	⅛ oz.	10
Blueberries, fresh	1 T.	8
Breadstick	1 piece	20
Broccoli	½ cup	14
Cantaloupe	1 piece (2 oz.)	4
Carrot	¼ cup	12
Cauliflower	½ cup	14
Cheese:		
American, imitation	1 oz.	70
Cheddar, imitation	1 oz.	90
Cottage	½ cup	110
Mozzarella, imitation	1 oz.	90
Swiss, imitation	1 oz.	80
Chow mein noodles	¼ cup	60
Coleslaw	½ cup	90
Crouton	1 piece	2
Cucumber	¼ cup	4
Mushroom	¼ cup	6
Onions, red	1 T.	4
Orange, fresh	1 piece	5
Pasta salad	½ cup	134
Peas, green	½ cup	60
Peaches, in syrup	1 piece	8
Peppers:		
Banana or mild pepperoncini	1 T.	18
Bell	¼ cup	4
Jalapeño	1 T.	9
Pineapple chunks in juice	½ cup	80
Tomato	1 oz.	6

Food and Description	Measure or Quantity	Calories
Turkey ham	¼ cup	46
Watermelon, fresh	1 piece (1 oz.)	1
Salad dressing:		
Regular:		
Blue cheese	1 T.	60
French, red	1 T.	70
Italian, golden	1 T.	45
Oil	1 T.	130
Ranch	1 T.	80
Thousand Island	1 T.	70
Dietetic:		
Bacon & tomato	1 T.	45
Cucumber, creamy	1 T.	50
Italian	1 T.	25
Thousand Island	1 T.	45
Wine vinegar	1 T.	2
Salad, Side, pick-up window	1 salad	110
Salad, taco	1 salad	390
Sausage	1 patty	200
Toast:		
Regular, with margarine	1 slice	125
French	1 slice	200
WESTERN DINNER, frozen:		
(Banquet) American Favorites	11-oz. dinner	513
(Morton) regular	11⅛-oz. dinner	347
(Swanson) *Hungry Man*	17½-oz. dinner	750
WHEATENA, cereal	¼ cup	112
WHEAT FLAKES CEREAL		
(Featherweight)	1¼ cups	100
WHEAT GERM CEREAL		
(Kretschmer)	¼ cup	110
WHEAT GERM, RAW (Elam's)	1 T.	28
WHEAT HEARTS, cereal		
(General Mills)	1 oz.	110
WHEATIES, cereal	1 cup	110
WHEAT & OATMEAL CEREAL,		
hot (Elam's)	1 oz.	105
WHISKEY SOUR COCKTAIL		
(Mr. Boston)	3 fl. oz.	120
***WHISKEY SOUR MIX**		
(Bar-Tender's)	3½ fl. oz.	177
WHITE CASTLE:		
Bun only	.9-oz. bun	74
Cheese only	1 piece	31
Cheeseburger	1 sandwich	200
Chicken sandwich	1 sandwich	186
Fish sandwich	1 sandwich	155
French fries	1 order	301
Hamburger	1 sandwich	161
Onion chips	1 order	329
Onion rings	1 order	245

Food and Description	Measure or Quantity	Calories
Sausage & egg sandwich	1 sandwich	322
Sausage sandwich	1 sandwich	196
WHITEFISH, LAKE:		
Baked, stuffed	4 oz.	244
Smoked	4 oz.	176
WIENER WRAP (Pillsbury)	1 piece	60
WILD BERRY DRINK,		
canned (Hi-C)	6 fl. oz.	88
WINCHELL'S DONUT HOUSE:		
Buttermilk, old fashioned	2-oz. piece	249
Cake, devil's food, iced	2-oz. piece	241
Cinnamon crumb	2-oz. piece	240
Iced, chocolate	2-oz. piece	227
Raised, glazed	1¾-oz. piece	212
WINE (See specific type, such as CHIANTI, SHERRY, etc.)		
WINE, COOKING (Regina):		
Burgundy or sauterne	¼ cup	2
Sherry	¼ cup	20
WINE COOLER (Bartles & Jaymes):		
Original white	6 oz.	92
Premium berry	6 oz.	92
Premium red	6 oz.	97

Y

Food and Description	Measure or Quantity	Calories
YEAST, BAKER'S (Fleischmann's):		
Dry, active	1 packet	20
Fresh & household, active	.6-oz. cake	15
YOGURT:		
Regular:		
Plain:		
(Bison)	8-oz. container	160
(Dannon):		
Low-fat	8-oz. cont.	110
Non-fat	8-oz. cont.	140
(Friendship)	8-oz. container	170
(Whitney's)	6-oz. container	150
Yoplait	6-oz. container	130
Plain with honey, *Yoplait, Custard Style*	6-oz. container	160
Apple:		
(Dannon) Dutch *Fruit-on-the-bottom*	8-oz. container	240
Yoplait	6-oz. container	190
Apple-cinnamon, *Yoplait, Breakfast Yogurt*	6-oz. container	240

Food and Description	Measure or Quantity	Calories
Apple & raisins (Whitney's)	6-oz. container	200
Apricot (Bison)	8-oz. container	262
Banana:		
(Dannon) *Fruit-on-the-bottom*	8-oz. container	240
LeShake (Kellogg's)	8-oz. container	170
Banana-Strawberry (Colombo)	8-oz. container	235
Berry (New Country) mixed	8-oz. container	210
Blueberry:		
(Bison):		
Regular	8-oz. container	262
Light	6-oz. container	162
(Breyer's)	8-oz. container	260
(Dannon) *Fresh Flavors*	8-oz. container	200
(New Country) supreme	8-oz. container	210
(Riché)	6-oz. container	180
(Sweet'N Low)	8-oz. container	150
(Whitney's)	6-oz. container	200
Yoplait	6-oz. container	190
Boysenberry:		
(Dannon)	8-oz. container	240
(Sweet'N Low)	8-oz. container	150
Cherry:		
(Breyer's) black	8-oz. container	270
(Dannon)	8-oz. container	240
(Friendship)	8-oz. container	230
(Riché)	6-oz. container	180
(Sweet 'n Low)	8-oz. container	150
Yoplait	6-oz. container	150
Cherry-vanilla (Colombo)	8-oz. container	250
Citrus, *Yoplait, Breakfast Yogurt*	6-oz. container	250
Coffee (Colombo; Dannon)	8-oz. container	200
Exotic fruit (Dannon)	8-oz. container	240
Fruit crunch (New Country)	9-oz. container	210
Guava (Colombo)	8-oz. container	240
Hawaiian salad (New Country)	8-oz. container	210
Honey vanilla (Colombo)	8-oz. container	220
Lemon:		
(Dannon) *Fresh Flavors*	8-oz. container	200
(New Country) supreme	8-oz. container	210
(Sweet'N Low)	8-oz. container	150
(Whitney's)	6-oz. container	200
Yoplait:		
Regular	6-oz. container	190
Custard Style	6-oz. container	180
Mixed berries (Dannon):		
Extra Smooth	4.4-oz. container	130
Fruit-on-the-Bottom	8-oz. container	240
Orange, *Yoplait*	6-oz. container	190
Orange supreme (New Country)	8-oz. container	210
Orchard, *Yoplait,*		
Breakfast Yogurt	6-oz. container	240

Food and Description	Measure or Quantity	Calories
Peach:		
(Bison)	8-oz. container	262
(Breyer's)	8-oz. container	270
(Dannon)	8-oz. container	240
(Friendship)	8-oz. container	240
(Meadow Gold) sundae style	8-oz. container	260
(New Country) 'n cream	8-oz. container	240
(Riché)	6-oz. container	180
(Sweet'N Low)	8-oz. container	150
(Whitney's)	6-oz. container	200
Peach melba (Colombo)	8-oz. container	230
Piña colada:		
(Dannon)	8-oz. container	240
(Friendship)	8-oz. container	230
Pineapple:		
(Breyer's)	8-oz. container	270
(Light n' Lively)	8-oz. container	240
Raspberry:		
(Breyer's) red	8-oz. container	260
(Dannon):		
Extra Smooth	4.4-oz. container	130
Fresh Flavors	8-oz. container	200
(Light n' Lively) red	8-oz. container	230
(Riché)	6-oz. container	180
(Sweet'N Low)	8-oz container	150
Yoplait:		
Regular	6-oz. container	190
Custard Style	6-oz. container	180
Raspberry ripple (New Country)	8-oz. container	240
Strawberry:		
(Breyer's)	8-oz. container	270
(Dannon) *Fresh Flavors*	8-oz. container	200
(Friendship)	8-oz. container	230
(Light n' Lively)	8-oz. container	240
(Meadow Gold)	8-oz. container	270
(Whitney's)	6-oz. container	200
Yoplait	6-oz. container	190
Strawberry-banana (Light n' Lively)	8-oz. container	260
Strawberry colada (Colombo)	8-oz. container	230
Tropical fruit (Sweet'N Low)	8-oz. container	150
Vanilla:		
(Breyer's)	8-oz. container	230
(Dannon):		
Fresh Flavors	8-oz. container	220
Hearty nuts & raisins	8-oz. container	270
(Friendship)	8-oz. container	210
(New Country) french ripple	8-oz container	240
(Whitney's)	6-oz. container	200
Yoplait, Custard Style	6-oz. container	180
Frozen, hard:		
Banana, *Danny-in-a-Cup*	8-oz. cup	210

Food and Description	Measure or Quantity	Calories
Boysenberry, *Danny-On-A-Stick,* carob coated	2½-fl.-oz. bar	140
Boysenberry swirl (Bison)	¼ of 16-oz. container	116
Cherry vanilla (Bison)	¼ of 16-oz. container	116
Chocolate:		
(Bison)	¼ of 16-oz. container	116
(Colombo) bar, chocolate coated	1 bar	145
(Dannon):		
Danny-in-a-Cup	8-fl.-oz. cup	190
Danny-On-A-Stick, chocolate coated	2½-fl.-oz. bar	130
Chocolate chip (Bison)	¼ of 16-oz. container	116
Chocolate chocolate chip (Colombo)	4-oz. serving	150
Mocha (Colombo) bar	1 bar	80
Piña colada:		
(Colombo)	4-oz. serving	110
(Dannon):		
(*Danny-in-a-Cup*	8-oz. cup	210
Danny-On-A-Stick	2½-fl.-oz. bar	65
Raspberry, red (Dannon):		
Danny-in-a-Cup	8-oz. container	210
Danny-On-A-Stick, chocolate coated	2½-fl.-oz. bar	130
Raspberry swirl (Bison)	¼ of 16-oz. container	116
Strawberry:		
(Bison)	¼ of 16-oz. container	116
(Colombo):		
Regular	4-oz. serving	110
Bar	1 bar	80
(Dannon):		
Danny-in-a-Cup	8 fl. oz.	210
Danny-Yo	3½ fl. oz.	110
Vanilla:		
(Bison)	¼ of 16-oz. container	116
(Colombo):		
Regular	4-oz. serving	110
Bar, chocolate coated	1 bar	145
(Dannon):		
Danny-in-a-Cup	8 fl. oz.	180
Danny-On-A-Stick	2½-fl.-oz. bar	65
Danny-Yo	3½-oz. serving	110
Frozen, soft (Colombo)	6-fl.-oz. serving	130
YOGURT DRINK (Dannon) *Dan'up*	8 oz.	190

Z

Food and
Description

Food and Description	Measure or Quantity	Calories
ZINFANDEL WINE (Inglenook)		
Vintage	3 fl. oz.	59
ZITI, FROZEN:		
(Morton) Light	11-oz. dinner	280
(Weight Watchers)	11¼-oz. meal	290
ZWEIBACK (Gerber: Nabisco)	1 piece	30